Queen Menopause

Queen Menopause

Finding your majesty in the mayhem

ALISON DADDO

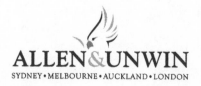

ALLEN&UNWIN
SYDNEY•MELBOURNE•AUCKLAND•LONDON

First published in 2022

Allen & Unwin
83 Alexander Street
Crows Nest NSW 2065
Australia
Phone: (61 2) 8425 0100
Email: info@allenandunwin.com
Web: www.allenandunwin.com

A catalogue record for this book is available from the National Library of Australia

ISBN 978 1 76087 539 8

Internal design by Bookhouse, Sydney
Set in 13.5/18.7 pt Fournier MT Std by Bookhouse, Sydney
Printed in Australia by McPherson's Printing Group

10 9 8 7 6 5 4 3 2

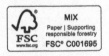

In celebration of women everywhere

Contents

Miserable magical menopause

The literature of menopause is the saddest, the most awful,
and the most medical of all genres. You're sleepless, you're
anxious, you're fat, you're depressed—and the advice is
always the same: take more walks, eat some kale, and drink
lots of water. It didn't help.

SANDRA TSING LOH

We live in a world where women are still mostly seen as
second class, where our beauty is our currency and our
aging bodies deem us somewhat invisible. Now that I'm well into
'middle age', I gratefully notice women who take exception to
becoming microscopic to the general public: women who fight
harder than most to continue to be hugely successful. I observe
these women as they battle stigma, harassment. Who are judged
not for what they say, the education and degrees they may hold,
but for what clothes they wear, how much weight they've gained
or lost, or how much grey is showing in their hair.

I also face this.

Women are powerful, especially as we get older, when we begin to care less about the external. We forget the society standard and turn our back on the beauty stamp of approval.

There are an incredible number of highly intelligent women I have been reading about for years. Women whose information, honesty, research, insights and wisdom I trust. I've shared pieces of their work throughout this book in the hope you may find some inspiration from them also.

Now that I've crossed that invisible line into menopause, into the second half of my life, I look around me in wonder . . . and sometimes despair.

It's a challenge to not see yourself the way your culture sees you. 'Past my prime', 'best years are behind me', etc., etc.

How did I get here so fast? For a long time, even as I was working at different jobs—as a birth assistant and teacher—I still wondered what I was going to be when I 'grew up'.

Guess what?

I'm here. I grew up. I also grew *out*. That seemed to happen fast too.

I wonder if that's important? Getting physically bigger. Perhaps I needed to take up more space in this world. Perhaps keeping small emotionally kept me small physically.

Maybe you are like me and are struggling with age and all its symptoms. Maybe you are also like me and are *so* sick and tired of the messages we receive about body shapes and wrinkles. Maybe you are also like me and are ready for a bigger, better second half of your life.

Writing this book goes against every fear I have about speaking my truth, having a strong opinion, being seen, and putting myself and my thoughts, words, actions on a platform to be analysed, dissected, judged.

I'm going to give it a whirl. I feel so challenged in all the varied places I have hidden away for so long.

Who am I to have a voice? Who am I not to?

But the cliff is there and I'm taking a leap. I don't think the cliff is that high, in all honesty. Maybe it's just a small step onto a bed of moss?

It's just all the machinations in my head. Let's do this.

Letter to you

Dear Reader,

I'm gathering you are here holding this book because you are about to experience or are on your path towards menopause.

This is what I want to say to you. There will be changes, both big and small. You can and will handle it all. When you look in the mirror and don't recognise your body anymore, when you feel angry all the time, or taken to the depths of despair, know that you are not alone, know that this is normal. *You* are normal. Know that millions of women have felt the same way as you. You might need to fight hard against the mood swings, take stock of your health, change your attitude towards your life, who you are, or who you *think* you are. Menopause might be the hardest battle of your life, but it might also be the best. It might even be the easiest transition ever. I believe in approaching menopause with a positive mindset, with a willingness to love yourself through the thick and thin of every symptom, and getting all the help you need. Choose—and by that I mean *really* make choices that don't seem like obvious ones—to find the positive in all that you are feeling. Find the healing. Step into the next phase of your life open to everything and anything. I believe that you, we, can all look back at this time in our lives and say, 'Now that was a ride'. You might have to drag yourself to the door of happiness and throw yourself in, but please, just do it. And see if you can drag your friends in with you. Collectively we are stronger, wiser and kinder. Be the light for other women who might need someone to show them that menopause is not the end. It's just the beginning.

Love,
Me

CHAPTER 1

So it begins . . .

I had other names for this book, such as,

Losing Your Eyebrows, Gaining a Beard
Death to Tampons!
Super Model to Super Old
Meno-What-the-Fuck?
Hell Hath No Fury Like a Woman Needing Chocolate
Why Can't You Read My Mind, You Complete Bastard?

If this book seems schizophrenic it's because *it is*. Different parts of my personality running amok, powered by hormones. You'll read my 'good days' and you'll read me at my worst and lowest days. That's my menopause. I've attempted to be as honest as I can, as I truly believe it's the only way to get through anything, especially anything that's challenging. And for me . . . that's menopause.

I needed to come back and rewrite the beginning of this book. This so-called 'adventure' of menopause keeps changing on me. Just when I think I have it figured out, I'm spun around 180 degrees and thrown another cartload of symptoms and feelings my way. It's also become a profound teacher. Teaching me about all the ways I kept myself small, quiet, ashamed, fearful of my power.

This is not your typical self-help book. There are times when I've been writing this book and I've been the one desperately needing help. I don't have all the answers. My life is not tied up in a perfect bow. What I do have is the desire to share the story of my experience with aging, menopause and self-love in the hope that it might resonate with you.

Menopause is an earthquake, shaking my internal organs, spine and joints, but most of all the depths of who I am. I'm now realising that this very well may be the whole *point* of menopause.

Who am I?

So, who am I to be talking about menopause?

Simply, a female who is traversing the highs and lows of this time in my life.

Some of you readers may remember me way back in the eighties and nineties as being a model, mostly known as a *Dolly* cover girl.

Menopause has me thinking a lot about what my 'story' is as a female.

As I look back on my life, I feel this through-line. A direct link between myself as a young girl who knew nothing about her body and the way it was changing and who I am now.

I remember the first terrifying moment of discovering my cycle had started, something I had no knowledge about. I hid my period from my mother. I felt ashamed and scared that I had it; there was no joy, celebration, no honour in becoming a young woman. I think, like a lot of girls of my generation and before me, I was led to believe that periods were hideous and painful. So, my periods were hideous and painful.

Surprise!

The changes to my cycle when entering perimenopause, and my hot flushes, were also something I had no idea about.

And, if society has its way, we are led to believe that not only is menopause also hideous and painful, like our periods, but that we shall not speak of it.

In making that link, I was determined to approach the end of my cycle, my fertility, in a different way to the beginning of it. I would not hide the fact I was in menopause; I would share what I was feeling and I would somehow celebrate the resolution of my cycle.

This has proved to be much harder than I first thought.

What follows is an account of some of the big moments that shaped who I am. The stepping stones that led me to some devastating experiences. The times I shrank inward and boarded up my heart, my hurt and my voice. I've had a lot of joy, love and fun also in my life. Though it's so often the painful experiences that shape and form how you operate in the world. In understanding me before menopause, I can understand the changes I want to make during and after menopause.

Puberty blues

I was horrified when my cycle started. All I had heard were the whispers from my older sisters and their friends about cramps and pimples every month. I had no clue about what or how to deal with my period. So when my cycle did start I hid my stained underwear from my mother. I remember thinking, this is *it*—I'm different now, I'm changed. I felt unclean and confused. I was embarrassed about my body and the changes that were afoot. Of course my mum eventually found my concealed underwear, and a packet of pads appeared on my chest of drawers the next day.

I began to manipulate my body, my emotions, to somehow feel like I 'fitted in'. Numbing my wisdom, my own advice, and my anger in case I seemed too much, crazy or stupid. You unconsciously know as a teenage girl there are unspoken rules, and like the good student I was, I followed them well.

Don't be confident.

Make sure you are pretty.

Don't sound like you're smart.

Don't be cocky.

Make sure other girls know you don't like your body.

But make sure you are in shape.

Make sure you are doing what others do so you can to be liked, but don't look like you are a copycat.

Etc. etc.

I'm sure patterns were playing themselves out before I hit my teens, though puberty, with all her magnifying feelings and emotions, turned the dial up to a ten. I was like millions of other little girls, including my mum and her mother before her: my period was an uninvited guest, it was here to stay, but by God she would not be welcomed or made to feel comfortable.

I had always been a people pleaser—I can't remember a time when I wasn't. People-pleasing was and still is today a familiar cloak of invisibility. If I'm liked, if I fit in, conform and be quiet, I'll get through, I'll pass without judgement.

Thirty-six years of stuffing down my words, compressing myself in big and small ways, is a long time. I was somewhat of an emotional pressure cooker, and ladies, let me tell you, if menopause has done one thing for me it has loosened my tongue and unleashed my anger, my words, my feelings, like nothing else before.

No wonder I'm burning up.

Modelling

I started modelling at the young age of sixteen. I'm the youngest of three sisters. I was the proverbial ugly duckling. Crazy-arse hair that no one, including my mum, could control. Huge eyes, a massive gap between my two front teeth, gangly body and a confidence level around one out of ten.

My view of myself as a young woman was still forming. Like a loose jelly in a cup I was easily pushed and pulled with no definitive direction. In so many ways the years I spent as a model shaped who I became and who I am today. I have often wanted to hide the fact I was a model. Run in the opposite direction of fame or beauty, because what was wrapped up in my modelling career was a lot of insecurity and fear. Modelling caused me to grow up in some ways very quickly because it gave me many opportunities a young woman rarely gets. At times it was an absolute blast.

I was 'discovered' at a party one day and sent off to an agency called Camerons (the name seemed to be my lucky sign; not only did I have a dog called Cameron, but I later married my soulmate with the same name).

I'm forever grateful I was sent to Camerons first, an agency run by the fabulous Jane Cameron. It was a kind and nurturing place for a young girl like myself.

I walked in with my one photo of myself from my year 10 formal and was immediately shuffled out the door for a Grace Bros catalogue casting. Shockingly, I booked the job.

I had been a dancer from ages five to fourteen, so having an awareness of my body and good posture lent itself to moving well in front of a camera.

Many times I had to do the old 'look like you're walking while not really walking' for the camera—creating the illusion of having a jaunty, devil-may-care stroll along the street. It was a case of hitting your mark while rocking back and forth, and while smiling, tossing your hair *and* looking like you're actually walking.

Truly, the similarities between brain surgery and modelling never cease to amaze me.

The next few years saw me in commercials, on magazine covers, as the face of the clothing brand Portmans, and hosting a children's game show.

Like so many Aussie teenage girls, I bought *Dolly* every month and followed the *Dolly* cover girl contest with great interest.

I even vaguely knew one of the winners because I'd competed against her in an athletics carnival in high school. She was, to me, a big celebrity.

The first time seeing myself on the pages of a magazine was so exciting. I was looking at myself in a way I'd never seen myself before. I can vividly remember the moment on a *Dolly* job I heard the words 'cover try'. What this meant was that during the shoot they would focus solely on taking photos for the cover of the magazine. Sometimes you would shoot a cover try and those photos were dismissed as not good enough. Sometimes you would see yourself front and centre on newsagents' stands. So, hearing those words made my heart skip a beat. Sure enough, that cover try made it and there I was, my first time on the cover. Surreal. I never dreamt that one day it would be me on the cover and so when that did eventuate it was delightful. Every *Dolly* cover I did I loved. I still love them all. I can see the progression of how I grew as a model from the first one to the last. And to be on so many covers was really special, and a great honour.

I took some amazing trips with *Dolly*, one of them being to the Greek islands. Usually it was a shoot down at Bondi or Tamarama Beach, including my first shoot with *Dolly*. But the Greece shoot will always remain special, as one of the most fun and hilarious shoots we ever did.

The *Dolly* team I worked with were a fun-loving, kind and energetic crew of women who knew what young girls like myself wanted to see and read about in a magazine. It was social media in magazine form, just better for your eyes and not so addictive.

So many women around my age still miss *Dolly* magazine; it defined our teens like nothing else.

Being a small part of the teenage-hood of many women my age is an honour. I know whenever I post an old photo from 'back in the day' I am flooded with messages of memories of that time and what *Dolly* meant to so many girls.

Becoming the 'Portmans girl' was another momentous experience.

I was one of the first models to land a contract that had me exclusively working for Portmans as a fashion label and no other. I would travel to Melbourne every three months or so and work with the amazing Angie Heinl; we had a great connection and the shoots were delightful to be on. Eventually the photo shoots became film commercials for Portmans, which Angie also directed. They were well received and brought a lot of joy. So much so that, with much delight, I later found out I had become a bit of a gay icon. The gay community would have Portmans parties and dress up and imitate my moves, most likely with Kylie Minogue blaring in the background.

Without modelling I may never have met my husband. He fell in love (or maybe lust) with an image of mine from a campaign for underwear called His Pants for Her. This was also shot by Angie. He would mention to me many months later, on our first date, that his crush on me was because of the His Pants for Her girl.

—

One of my most beloved modelling stories is my pirate, turtle eggs, deserted island account.

Here goes . . .

I was booked for an Alpine cigarette print shoot; not sure if you remember those—they always involved a smiling woman and sometimes man, dressed all in white, on a white sandy beach with turquoise water swirling around their ankles. They never actually had a cigarette in their hands; it symbolised the 'lifestyle' of what a cigarette can give you, I guess. Because nothing says 'buy cigarettes' like two healthy-looking people frolicking on a gorgeous beach.

The shoot was set for Malaysia. Myself, the male model, makeup artist, photographer and assistant all arrived in Kuala Lumpur and drove through beautiful scenery to a seaside town, to stay at a Club Med. Only trouble was the sand at Club Med was not pure white and the water was not turquoise.

So, after phoning around, and talking to locals, a fishing boat was hired to take us to a deserted island where such things could be found.

That boat trip to the island was crazy. The boat had to be 60 years old and the two fishermen at least 90 in the shade. Halfway there, with no land in sight, the boat broke down and we started taking on water. Buckets were used to toss out seawater and finally the motor started once more and on we travelled.

Three hours later we arrived at the most stunning little island I've ever seen. And lo and behold, it had all the elements the shoot desired . . . white sand, turquoise water.

Makeup was applied, white sarong and bikini popped on and away we went—let the frolicking begin.

As we had lost so much time travelling between the mainland and the island, the shoot was not finished once we started losing the light. So, the idea was, we would sleep on the beach overnight, finish the shoot the next morning, and hightail it back with our Malay fishermen the next day.

We were fortunate that the island was a fisherman's paradise; there was a deck with rudimentary cover over it and some camp-style beds out in the open. Two spearfishermen walked up and out of the water like a miracle and thankfully shared their catch with us, which to this day is some of the most incredible seafood I've ever tasted.

We lay down on the camp beds with full bellies listening to the sound of the wild monkeys that inhabited the island.

Awoken sometime later by the spearfishermen, we were alerted that an enormous green sea turtle was on the beach laying her eggs. Flashlights in hand, we carefully approached her and watched her lay hundreds of eggs. As we were marvelling at this beautiful scene, our spearfishing friends turned the flashlights off and immediately told us to hide in the jungle. They had spotted a pirate ship just off the coast. These pirates would come looking for the turtle eggs to sell at market. At the time they were worth between one to two dollars an egg; that's quite a haul back then when you are talking at least 200 eggs from just one turtle. Pirates were known to kill anyone they thought might be in their way of collecting the 'treasure'. So into the jungle we ran, hiding behind palm trees. It was a sad time, knowing all those eggs were stolen; they left not a single one to start the cycle of life again.

Needless to say, once the pirates left, we all finally had some sleep, finished the shoot the next morning, and made our way back to the mainland with our fishermen friends. Quite the adventure.

With modelling I learned you often had to let go and go with the flow, as they say. The easier I could make the job for everyone, the better the photos and the more fun the experience.

I know that while my image came across as a joyful, carefree, relatable, pretty young thing, there was a flip side, too—not to say that all those elements were not there as well. I was grateful to be in the position I was, I worked hard and I had a joyous time for so many of my modelling days, but there was a dark side. And so when it came time to say goodbye to modelling, it was easy for me.

I don't regret becoming a model. Regretting that time in my life would not serve me in any shape or form. I was incredibly fortunate to work and make friends with some lovely fashion editors, makeup artists, agents and photographers. The money was good, and the travel was amazing. Japan, London, Spain, and more.

There were some exciting adventures, ones that I never would have had, had I not entered the world of fashion.

On paper and from the outside it all sounds glamorous. And it can be.

What it can also be is degrading, dangerous, exhausting and it can batter your self-confidence to a pulp.

I was hurtling through life semi-conscious of who I was and what I was doing, and modelling swept me up in such a way that I was at times unaware of what was happening around me. It's an industry that, to state the obvious, only cares about how you look. Beginning and end of sentence. Being loved for an image that is portrayed on the front of a magazine is a fragile and thin form of admiration and most certainly has a time limit.

I didn't recognise that I had a choice to speak up when something was uncomfortable or when I was in any sort of pain on the job. I was a shy sixteen-year-old and I was mostly surrounded by older people. Your job is not to give opinions and speak your mind. Your job is to look pretty and make the clothes/makeup/ ice-cream/products look fabulous.

I had an incident very early in my career when on a job, after a request from the fashion editor for my hair to be in curly ringlets for the shoot. I sat quietly in the hair and makeup chair as my scalp and the tops of my ears were burned and blistered by a curling iron wielded by a coked-out hair stylist.

To this day if I ever see those bloody curling tongs I want to declare war and break them with a sharp object.

I was sixteen. I didn't feel I had a voice to say 'enough'. I just grinned (with tears in my eyes) and bared it. All the while my hair and scalp were going up in smoke.

I remember not knowing how to move in front of the camera that day, with my head screaming in pain and feeling more than a little shellshocked.

I'm sure my face showed how I was feeling. The photographer didn't care; he only cared that he got the shot.

I don't know how many others were taking drugs that day. Pretty sure it was most of the crew. I only know it was a nightmare.

I don't remember letting my agency know of my experience. I wouldn't have wanted to rock the boat or create a fuss.

What I did do was tell my dad.

A bunch of flowers arrived at my house the next day with an apology from the magazine. It wasn't until years later, well after I'd given modelling away, that I found out my dad had in fact made a massive fuss.

To my agent, the magazine and the photographer.

Dad was a high court magistrate at the time and not a person to be messed with.

I believe there were some pretty choice words with the terms 'legal action' and 'the photographer will never work again' thrown around.

I love him for that.

Never once on that shoot did I feel I could have walked out the door or stood up for myself. I stayed silent.

On another job, another hair stylist who was having a bad day told me I had hair like Queen Elizabeth (odd slur, I know, that now makes me giggle), whacked me in the head with his hairbrush and walked off the set.

Fun!

Countless swimsuit shoots at 6 a.m. on winter mornings and being told to 'think warm'. Being discussed like an object while in full earshot.

Haircuts on the job that were atrocious, and breasts gaffer-taped together to give me a cleavage.

One music video I did in London had me inside a warehouse at 2 a.m., balancing on a metal girder in a construction zone built for the video. I was handed an electric grinder used for cutting through metal so they could have those 'sparks flying' while I danced to the pre-recorded song.

Think Jennifer Beals in *Flashdance*, right?

Surprisingly, I had never handled a grinder before. I know you must be shocked, an eighteen-year-old girl still not up on how to cut through large sheets of metal.

Travesty.

I was wearing cut-off shorts and a tank top. No mask, and to top it off the construction site was flooded with water. Because it gave a great 'effect' for filming.

The crew were all standing 20 feet away on dry land as they said they were 'afraid of being electrocuted'.

But, I did the job. I danced with the metal grinder, made some sparks fly, smiled like it was the most fun, 2 a.m. thing I'd ever done, and then got the hell out of there before they handed me a chainsaw and asked me to cut down a telegraph pole.

The song was never released.

So, the video . . . well who knows where the video is?

~

There was sexual harassment both large and small.

My first job working for a magazine, still only sixteen and a virgin. While standing in front of the camera the photographer wanted to know if I'd had sex with my boyfriend.

'What was it like?' Asking me these questions and more in front of a full crew of people. I didn't know it was sexual harassment at the time.

Again, I didn't say a word to anyone—family, friends or my agent. I thought it was something I had to just put up with, go along with, in order to be a model.

I put up and shut up and did what I was told, not just for work, but in just about every situation that came my way.

Oh man, if I could go back in time and protect my young naive self from the mishaps I had. Now, as a mother, if my children were ever in the same situation, just the thought of them being treated in such ways makes my blood boil.

Clearly the common denominator here is feeling like I didn't have a voice. I didn't even realise I *should* be angry at the questions and treatment I was receiving. I didn't know I needed to protect myself and draw a strong, clear boundary. Thankfully, age has taught me how to do this very thing with gusto.

At one point I had the proverbial 'carrot' dangling perilously close to my face. I travelled to London when I was eighteen and was represented by an agency called Storm. I remember heading out to casting calls with a bunch of other young models from the same agency and every now and then a young girl in her school uniform would appear as well.

She was cute, shorter than me, which was unusual as I was always on the shorter side of the typical model height. I never imagined that this young, skinny schoolgirl would go on to become Kate Moss the supermodel.

I stayed in London for about a year, had moderate success with work, then went home to Australia for a few months and travelled back to London again and stayed almost another year. Eventually

I left again as my sister was getting married and I wanted to go home to be her bridesmaid.

I knew I was leaving for good.

Word from my London agent was that I was about to 'blow up' like Kate Moss when I left. Would I? Who knows. I don't regret not going back. Though I do wonder what would have happened had I stayed. Would I have risen to dizzying heights like Kate Moss? I think not, but I might have had a few more exciting opportunities and travelled a lot more. As I watched Kate's career explode I was on my way to L.A. and already heading towards quitting the industry.

I wasn't a particularly ambitious model. I knew it wasn't my future; I was on a fast-moving train and simply hung on.

As I look back at that time in my life I wonder, in hindsight, would I do anything differently?

First and foremost, I would have stayed in school and graduated. Started modelling at eighteen or twenty, once I had bit more sense under my belt. I don't know why I was in such a rush, I must have felt like I had enough knowledge and was mature enough at sixteen to handle everything that would come my way.

The excitement and allure of modelling called to me louder than school at the time. Basically, my young mind could not have imagined what I would need to deal with. I was offered an opportunity and I jumped. Being young and naive I thought I would skip some school and make a little money. I got way more than I bargained for. I'm still glad I gave modelling the time and energy I did.

It doesn't take the modelling industry to be sexually harassed or find ourselves in awkward, horrible situations that we put up with and fake smile our way through. In any profession many women do exactly the same thing I did.

Japan

One event from my past has irrevocably changed who I am. The experience exemplifies my realisation of not feeling entitled to my own safety. It's not easy to write, or speak about. I've added it here to give the experience breathing room. To see the words on paper and tell my story, because I know for sure that some of you reading will have your own experience of being sexually assaulted. How it shaped me as a woman, how I straddle the breadth of my sensual self, my self-image and depths of self-hatred, are all tied up in this experience.

I have spent many hours with a therapist and friends exploring and processing what happened to me, which is why I feel I can share this now, from a place of holding the assault with tender care. If this story stirs you because you yourself have dealt with sexual assault, firstly, I am so sorry for what you went through, and, secondly, I want you to find someone to talk about it with. Someone who can hold you, hear you and work through all the feelings that may come along with your experience. A ghost from the past can hinder so many things in the future.

I was only seventeen when I was asked if I'd consider modelling in Japan. Japan was full of Western models all looking to earn money on a two-month contract.

The Japanese fashion industry loved models that were 'cute'-looking. I fell under that category at the time and so was offered a two-month contract to live and work in Tokyo by a Japanese modelling agency.

Without much thought, other than a pleading chat with my parents about leaving school halfway through year 11, I said yes.

I was a young, non-streetwise girl. I don't think I'd ever made myself more than a frozen pizza for dinner, or done my own laundry.

I ventured out into the big, wide world blindly.

I was in a foreign country; everything was so different—the culture, the language, food, the public transport, and the way the modelling industry operated. It was nothing for me to be doing three jobs in one day, seven days a week.

I was living in what could be called the model barracks. Tiny one-room apartments that, to be honest, I barely spent any time in due to my workload.

There were other models living in the apartment block with me, though we were pretty much ships in the night, or mostly tired ships passing in the early hours of the morning.

I had reached the halfway mark of my contract and was fortunate enough to be paired up with an English model called Sybil on quite a few jobs. We struck up a friendship. Most of the girls in Japan were on their own, wide-eyed and patchworking their days together with work, clubs at night, sleep and more work.

Finding a friend in a foreign city was a breath of fresh air.

Sybil invited me to a party she'd heard was being hosted at some model's apartment. I was excited. Every other night was spent in my tiny room with a pot of rice or packet of noodles attempting to reach my family or my boyfriend on the rotary phone in my room.

I pulled on my ripped-at-the-knees, 1980s high-waisted jeans, wrapped a black leather belt tight around the belt loops. Threw on my long-sleeved black T-shirt that was short enough to show a slice of my belly, and met Sybil for our night out.

Entering, it was like any other party: beers, loud music, groups of people laughing and shouting to be heard over the music.

As neither of us knew anyone else there, Sybil and I stuck together. About 30 minutes into the party, we were sitting on a couch talking when two unknown guys ran towards us. They physically picked me up and shoved me into the closet that was part of the room where the party was taking place. I was groped, flesh twisting, tongues shoved into my unwelcome mouth. In the space of being held in the closet I was fighting to get out, calling for help. I remember seeing flashes of people unaware—dancing, drinking. And then, nothing. They were pulled from my flailing body by another guy. An unknown hero who said, 'Enough, let her up.' It was then that one of them uttered, 'If she's going to dress like that, she was asking for it.'

Jeans and a T-shirt?

I was in shock, disbelief, at what had just taken place: one minute enjoying the company of a friend, the next rescued from a closet by a stranger. As I stood there in the aftermath, I don't know what I did exactly. All I know was I felt immediately mortified and embarrassed. The knight in shining armour offered to get me home, which I gladly accepted.

We talked on the way, taking the train and walking back. He told me he was a professional boxer from America and a model. He was kind, funny, and I was grateful to have an escort home.

Upon reaching my small room he asked to come in, and I felt like I couldn't say no. I opened the door and in he stepped. What took place next is a confusing mess.

He forced himself on me, and I said 'No'. He cajoled, he pushed more. I still said 'No'. 'I have a boyfriend,' I pleaded. Again, I said 'No'. He pushed me back on the unmade bed I'd hurriedly left just hours before. I said 'No'. I was utterly terrified. Once his body was on top of mine, once his arms gripped mine, once I was unable to move, I gave in. I let the rape happen.

Once he was gone, I showered and cried, and I totally panicked. I knew that I could tell no one of what took place. I must have led him on. I had somehow cheated on my boyfriend, hadn't I? I felt sick to my stomach, and so much shame.

So, for the longest time I held the experience as a secret— a dirty secret. I compartmentalised the rape. Hiding it away like a locked-up box shoved under my bed.

I fully believed that it was my fault.

I had let him walk me home, I said yes to him coming into my apartment; he had saved me, hadn't he?

I wanted the experience buried and gone.

I had also not fought back. I caved in to this man as I was terrified of what he could do to me, so I let him do whatever he wanted. So, in my mind, it couldn't have been rape.

Today he remains nameless and faceless, a dark-haired shadow man from America.

It wasn't until some twelve years later in therapy when I shared my experience for the very first time that I fully understood the extent of what I went through.

In finally putting words to my experience with a therapist, someone who cared, I was able to shift my perception of the rape from being my fault to understanding I was the victim.

Up until then, the weight of blaming myself was constant. I remember my therapist telling me how smart I was to not fight back, as the man was a professional boxer and I may have ended up with a lot more than self-hatred.

I did come out of it physically unharmed, which is more than most women, yet the idea of not fighting back was deeply linked to a cesspool of shame.

Living with shame is a slow and painful way to rob you of self-love and compassion for yourself. It was a poison to my soul, and only continued to cement my deep insecurity about being worthy of anyone's love.

The experience changed the way I felt about myself as a female and about my sexuality. Being too sexy was dangerous. Being a female meant I could be yanked from my life, broken and used up like a dirty dishrag. Being a female, I had better be so careful about how I speak to people, especially men: make less eye contact, make sure I wasn't putting out any 'signals'. Dress down, be smaller, be invisible.

Which was the antithesis of the career I was building as a model!

For years I never felt anger at those young men, all three of them and what they did. I entombed that, along with the whole experience.

All I felt was guilt and disgust with myself.

Too many times we as women do not own our anger. I certainly had not owned my anger. My righteous anger.

We are deemed bitchy, crazy, hormonal, difficult, and all the while what we are truly feeling is bloody furious.

With two daughters of my own, I want them to own every ounce of their anger. It's imperative. And as for my son, yes, of course have your anger, though make sure you have your tears, your vulnerability, your heart.

All while their mum is still undoing the shackles and binds that still to this day can hold my anger in check.

There are days when I still feel I'm recovering from being a model. Days when I want to not care that my body and face have aged, that once the camera who 'loved me' now seems to want to make my nose look enormous and add droopy bags under my eyes.

We live in the world of selfies, where a large majority of Instagram content is people selfie-ing themselves in all sorts of locations and at all kinds of events, even if the event is as riveting as eating a peanut butter sandwich. Selfies and me are currently not friends.

I've attempted this strange new trend myself, though I'm always horrified as to how they turn out. It's like there is some sort of code, or angle or filter (oh, those filters can be a dangerous thing). Bravo to those who have mastered the art. I don't know how women and girls do it so well.

Honestly, though, why the hell should I care?

Some days I look in the mirror and love what I see, love how I feel, the strength returning to my body now that it's moving again, the lines on my face caused by laughter and smiles.

Simply grateful that my body is (mostly) working as it should.

After living in America for 25 years and pursuing careers that were far from the entertainment industry and staying out of the public eye, there have been times since moving back to Australia I've felt uncomfortable being recognised from an old *Dolly* mag.

I feel embarrassed, as if somehow I might let that woman down with the way I look now. Their childhood pin-up girl—now a mother with arm flaps and dodgy knees.

This is one of the surprising impacts from modelling in those young years that has stayed with me long past the time when *Dolly* magazines were packed away in a plastic box to grow mould in a garage.

I know the modelling industry is a tantalising topic. There are stories to tell for sure. Good, bad and ugly tales from long ago.

I did not spend my formative years being a strong, confident outspoken woman. But here I am, halfway through my life, with a determination that I will always have my own back, and speak up when I feel threatened. I have earned my wisdom through experience and there is no better time than now to fully own it.

Marriage and moving

Life took an unexpected turn when meeting my 'crush', a Mr Cameron Daddo, at the age of twenty. Cam was a big heartthrob at the time: the youngest game show host in the history of Aussie TV, he had gone on to have a hugely successful musical theatre and TV career.

I'd been a fan since the age of sixteen, watching him all dewy eyed as he hosted *Perfect Match*. One of the bonuses of working with *Dolly* magazine was meeting Carlotta Moye, then a fashion editor (now one of Australia's top fashion photographers). We quickly became great friends. I credit her with much of my success as a model as she booked me continuously through those years, hence the multiple *Dolly* covers.

Carlotta was also the reason Cam and I met.

Cam was at *Dolly* one day and happened to make a compliment about one of my photos on the wall. Carlotta, knowing my not-so-secret crush on Cam, called me immediately to let me know he had been in the office and would I like her to help us meet each other. There was a party my friend was throwing that weekend at a nightclub. Cam was invited. While waiting for him to arrive I had a few too many vodkas for some Dutch courage. He walked in and my knees went weak. I attempted to act cool and failed miserably. The vodka made my nerves worse, so I ended up making absurd comments that unfortunately now live in infamy within the 'first time we met' storyline. My husband's memory is ridiculously good from the 1990s; he has trouble remembering things from yesterday but that moment, and what we said, he remembers word for bloody word.

We spoke for a while, and he invited me out on a date the next day. Bob's your uncle and Shirley's your aunt.

That was *it*. Crazy, mad, love.

Two and a half months later, we were engaged. One year after that, we were married.

Eight months from our wedding day I had my 23rd birthday in Los Angeles, having packed our bags and dreams and moved so Cam could give Hollywood a good shake.

I was horrified about moving to L.A. I had an unfair idea about what America was going to be like. Too many *Charlie's Angels* and *Hill Street Blues* episodes portrayed America as a place of gang violence, car chases and inedible food. I had a booming career in Australia, family, and a deep love of my country. I'd sworn I'd never live anywhere else.

Cam announced we were moving, whether I wanted to or not. He had an opportunity he needed to jump on and he was leaving to make his fame and fortune and dreams come true.

So, in following the theme of my life, I didn't fight the decision. I felt there was no other choice but to go, as devastated as I was.

Remember: we were 22 and 26—young, naive and unable to communicate in a way that was equal and thoughtful.

Oh Lord, were we babes in the woods. September of 1991, we landed in L.A.

It was hot and smelly, and my first meal lived up to my expectations of inedible food. (Thankfully, more time spent opened my eyes to the joy, fun and yumminess of living there.)

Modelling in L.A. was never going to work for me; the age of Pamela Anderson and *Baywatch* was upon America, especially in California, and I was still a fairly skinny, flat-chested, not so tall, crazy-haired gal from Sydney.

I was asked repeatedly by my L.A. agent if I would consider breast implants. I had gone from an Aussie covergirl, to an inadequate, need-to-be-fixed/changed face in the crowd. I was a nobody in L.A. No friends, no career—a fish out of water.

The day I decided to wave bye bye to modelling was joyous, because my new career as a mother was in sight and I could not wait. My tyres left skid marks on the road as I drove away from the agency for the last time. I never looked back.

Therapy

While my marriage was a happy one for a few years, I always had a tiny fear at the back of my mind that Cam would leave me for someone better. Someone smarter, sexier, more talented, more beautiful. He was the handsome Aussie heartthrob that many women were in love with. In my mind he could have the pick of any woman he wanted. I worried that one day he would pick someone other than me.

We both had been floundering our way through all the trials and tribulations of marriage, moving countries and careers. It was inevitable that we would fall apart. I think a part of me expected it to happen. We were just so young. Moving to America and not knowing a soul placed a lot of pressure on the marriage. Cam was pushing hard with auditions and gaining work here and there. I was a bit lost and terribly lonely and relied on Cam for much of my happiness.

My world splintered when we separated. Hopes and dreams came crashing down around me. I couldn't fathom being with anyone else. I couldn't dream of anyone else that I wanted to be a parent with.

Seeking therapy for our marriage was by far the best life decision I've ever made. Because it's here that I was able to begin making sense of who I was and what I needed to heal.

Months and months of therapy lay ahead of me. I was miserable yet determined to understand myself and why I continued to choose the same type of men and create the same relationships.

It's a long, detailed story about the coming back together of our marriage.

I am forever grateful that we went through that experience, that we chose to stay and dig deep into who we were. That we chose love over fear.

We both did therapy; we both knew we were still in love and we both knew we needed to change.

I could write about every nuance of grief and pain, of which there were plenty, but it would be an injustice to who we are now *because* of the fracture in our marriage.

And the universe knew too, knew that there was a better road ahead, a better life, if we were brave enough to take it. To fall down and get up time and time again. Hang in there when times were tough. And they were. I was leaving Cam almost every week. Some days I could not bear to see his face. Slowly but surely, over a year, the healing happened.

It changed the dynamic of our marriage for the better, it hurt like hell and tapped into my deepest insecurities, and it helped me grow so much I'll be forever grateful. The fertile mud of your life.

Now 30 years later—30 years of loving the same guy—we still call upon the tools we learned in therapy to manoeuvre our way through any challenging time. Right now, with menopause and hormones raging, our marriage has gone through some serious tests. Remembering communication—being brave, being open and being vulnerable with each other—has proven to never fail in creating the intimacy we both crave. Even while I've wanted to run away with the circus.

The pain and hurt created during that time also actualised the best soil to grow the most exquisite flower our little world had ever seen.

Within a year of living apart and counselling, we renewed our vows. A week before the renewal ceremony I had found out I was pregnant with our daughter Lotus.

Thankfully, our lives and marriage would be infinitely happier.

Full circle

In May 1996 our first of three amazing children were born. Fifty-six hours of labour, and Lotus arrived.

Nothing had prepared me for the joy and love I would feel when our baby girl was placed in my arms. Nothing prepared me for the swollen breasts, lack of sleep, hormonal emotional rollercoaster and the fear of feeling I was not capable of raising and caring for a baby. I'd read *What to Expect When You're Expecting*, wasn't that enough? (Rolling of the eyes is completely necessary here.)

I was *so* naive.

What shocked me about becoming pregnant more than anything was the number of negative reactions I received. The horror stories of pregnancy and birth gone wrong. The sleepless nights and strain on the marriage.

There was so little of the miracle of birth, the joy, the feeling of unconditional love.

I was still working with our counsellor, Doreen. I shared my feelings and concerns about the negativity that surrounds women in childbirth.

Doreen recognised my love and passion for the birthing process and I was offered the opportunity to come and work and train under her through The Bodyful Mind Institute.

My work allowed me an in-depth perspective of working with couples before the baby is born, creating a safe and loving environment for the birth and dealing with any fears and concerns that either of them may have had. Basically, creating as clear a path for the newborn as possible.

I eventually became the Director of Pregnancy and Family Development. I studied for my massage therapist licence so I could use that skill for pregnant mums and newborn babies.

Attending births has been a miracle, all the births—from home to hospital. Each one is as special as the last. I am forever changed and grateful that I was allowed into the lives of the families to assist in supporting bringing their babies into this world.

Through my work with women and birth I feel a deep connection to menopause. Witnessing the next stage of women's lives as they birth themselves as a mother. And now, witnessing not only myself but others change gears again and birth something new within themselves through menopause.

The cycle of life; how life-changing both childbearing and menopause can be.

Speaking up

I've learned over the years that expressing myself clearly and honestly when it comes to matters *other* than myself is pretty easy. Growing up, my self-expression was minimal. Especially anything to do with my intimate feelings. I didn't know anyone who did speak honestly and openly about feelings.

Tell my parents I was scared or lonely? What a concept! Kids are amazing at creating emotional pockets for their feelings. I know I had bulging ones.

After seeking therapy for our marriage breakdown and enjoying the process of unfolding and unpacking so many hidden feelings, I joined group therapy. I was surrounded by kind, thoughtful people who were open and willing to share in front of others. And most importantly, who wanted to listen to me. I was challenged by this. Having only really begun to express myself to my therapist, the idea of a larger audience terrified me.

I was incredibly fortunate to be a part of the group I was in. It was here I began to trust my feelings, and began to coax my scared little voice into sharing who I was and wanted to be.

Telling my story with compassionate ears listening was so healing and important for me.

Hearing others tell their story, learning from them through their communication of thoughts and actions remains to this day my favourite way to connect with another human being.

Storytelling has been the human way of handing down wisdom since time began. I sometimes wonder with the invention of computers and the iPhone whether we are losing the art of face-to-face communication.

During my younger years and to this day writing in a journal has enabled me to understand myself better. I have filled multiple journals in my life, each of them a treasure and as important as the next.

I know talking about menopause is not for every woman, but if you feel like you want to open up and share, I'll bet you'll find many of us out there ready and willing to share our stories with you and listen to yours.

It's good for the soul.

Finally speaking about all the things big and small that I needed to get off my chest was and continues to be a lifesaver.

When I first began to share my feelings about beginning perimenopause, I could feel the restraints around this topic. Did I even want to admit I was in perimenopause? It's not like saying I was pregnant—no one burst into tears of joy and congratulated me. Small outfits were not knitted and presented with joy. As for baby showers, now it was more like a glass of wine (with lots of ice) and some tissues. That's about as much of a celebration most women get.

What was *my* belief about menopause?

I never even thought about it before I had symptoms. I didn't care much to read anything because it sounded like a train wreck ahead of me. I was secretly thinking, 'I'm healthy, I'm a positive person, I eat well, menopause will be a breeze. I probably won't even get it till I'm in my sixties. I don't need to be worrying or thinking about it.' It was something that happened to old women, I thought. I was young, right?

I certainly never *asked* any women, including my mum, about menopause.

The society we live in speaks loudly about aging in general and menopause is part of that category. Pretty much it's, 'Your body is about to change for the worse', 'Get ready for sleepless nights', 'Sex is over', or 'You'll be fat and depressed'.

To name a few. Yippee!

We know that in regards to advertising, aging isn't something that's been lifted up and complimented. It's been about how to *stop* the aging process, even before you bloody well get to what's considered old.

Women over 40 are huge consumers of products, and yet where is the representation of us in the media?

It's enough to put frown marks on my frown marks.

No, menopause is not the 'cutest' of subjects. It's not the most thrilling of dinner conversations, or the best small talk over the copy machine with your male co-workers. But it sure is necessary.

Letter to my twenty-year-old self

Dear Ali,

You were cute, cuter than you thought. You were also floating two feet above the ground most of the time. Find something that grounds you. Stop looking outside yourself for love. You are enough. Stay out of the sun. Invest in property! You are never going to please everyone. You are never going to be happy trying to please everyone. Remember, you can say *No*. Don't worry about feeling stupid, okay? You'll learn a whole lot of stuff in the next 30 years. Trust me, you'll live through some heavy shit and you'll take notes. Ask your mum about her life, her menopause; in fact, ask a lot of people. Be ready, be kinder to yourself. Go for your dreams.

Allow your anger to be owned and spoken. Trust your instincts. Don't let anybody else define who you are.

Love,
Me

I don't want to be accepted. I want to be loved. If you have the choice between love or acceptance, which would you pick?

Sonya Renee Taylor
....

CHAPTER 2

What is menopause?

M y greatest joy is spending time with other women and sharing stories and life experiences. It leaves me feeling that I am not alone. As they say, 'a problem shared is a problem halved'.

I believe we need to talk about menopause; we need to talk about how we are feeling about it all—the loss of our period/ fertility.

What all of this means to *us*.

We need to, because there is a slippery slope of somehow feeling that menopause is the death of something—our femininity, our womanliness. I'm throwing down my hand-held, battery-operated fan and saying, HELL NO.

I want to use menopause as a beginning. Mother Nature can't be wrong, right?

She can't have created us to hit a midlife number and expect us to lie down and be done with life, fun, sex, feeling good.

After years of taking care of others it seems that many of us have forgotten how to dream and tap into what our deepest desires truly are.

So begins my deep dive into menopause. Why do we have menopause?

Yeah, I get the Dr Biological reason, but *why*? What are we being called to do? To feel? To become?

With those questions, I've started talking with other women about how menopause has changed them, and how they embraced the physical and emotional elements of this time. Like, what has changed for the better for them? Has their relationship evolved? Has their femininity changed at all through menopause?

As I write this, I'm still waking through the night lying in a pool of sweat or being driven mad by the sound of my husband chewing so much that I need to exit the room in a mad rush.

That's all still real for me.

What is happening to our bodies?

Until I started researching, I didn't know the exact science of why, when and wtf. I'll break it down into simple terms.

There are three stages:

1. perimenopause
2. menopause
3. postmenopause.

Perimenopause

Periods begin to change as the production of progesterone and oestrogen slows down. During the decline of those two hormones we are in perimenopause. That's when you'll probably notice a change in your cycle. This stage usually lasts anywhere from four to eight years.

Perimenopause is often the most challenging time as you may be having symptoms for multiple years. You may also be in perimenopause and not even realise it! Skipping periods or an unusually heavy flow might be your first symptom. Breast tenderness is another common symptom. You might experience some body aches and pains. You may feel like you did when you were first pregnant. Twice I bought a home pregnancy test thinking that I might be pregnant. Remember you can still get pregnant in perimenopause, even if your cycle is shifting. When I check in with other women about the length of time they were in perimenopause I get so many differing answers—five years, ten years.

Having a blood test to check your hormones will confirm if you have begun perimenopause. This is when you may swing anywhere between having no symptoms to having crazy wild symptoms.

Menopause

The term menopause refers to the time after your final menstrual cycle and the year that then follows. Ovulation no longer occurs and production of oestrogen and progesterone ceases. The average

age for women to reach menopause is usually between the ages of 45 and 55 years.

Once you recognise you are well into perimenopause, start tracking your cycle so you know the date of your last cycle.

I've been fooled twice now thinking I was in menopause as I'd not had a period for many months, then *boom*, along came my period. I needed to start counting again from that day on to know exactly when menopause did begin. It's all fun and games. ☺

Symptoms may stay the same as for perimenopause or you may have a few new ones to call your own; a change of skin and hair might be something that comes along at this point.

Postmenopause

The final stage is postmenopause. Once you have gone at least a year without a period you are postmenopausal. Symptoms will ease. Fireworks explode in the sky, the Queen grants you a public holiday and Oprah Winfrey gives you a new car.

Sleeping naked in winter will become a thing of the past, unless you enjoy it. Your body settles down from all the changes.

You've been through a lot in these past years—take some time to check in with your doctor, as getting an extra boost for your bones and heart at this stage is a great idea.

It may be difficult to know exactly when menopause officially ends. When are you postmenopausal? Is there a knock at the door with a huge bunch of flowers, confetti and a lifetime supply of chocolate? Do you start to actually sleep all through the night?

Apparently the answer is basically, yes, the symptoms begin to wane, and most women might experience the joy of sleeping easily through the night again. You feel more like you again, the brain fog lifts and you can no longer light a candle and the bed sheets with one of your hot flushes. The mood swings become more balanced. Some women do continue to experience hot flushes years after their period stops, but by that stage a hot flush here and there is not even a blip on the screen. There might be lingering symptoms that will need to be addressed continually for others.

But mostly, you have passed through the Southern Oracle, survived the Sphinx opening its laser eyes and are now free to walk into the remainder of your lovely life. Or, as it might also be called, *The NeverEnding Story*?

What are the symptoms that tell us perimenopause is on its way?

For the majority of women, symptoms of menopause or perimenopause begin well before your periods come to an end. All the changes you are experiencing are from your hormones becoming unbalanced. There may be other underlying health issues also, so it's best to see your doctor and talk about any challenges you might be facing.

Okay, so here's THE LIST. You may end up with none of these, or only a few. My eyes bulged a little when I first read what was possibly in store for me. DO NOT PANIC. There's a lot of help out there! Some of the most 'exciting' ones are:

- difficulty concentrating
- hot flushes

- mood swings
- trouble sleeping or broken sleep
- brain fog, lapses in memory
- dry hair or skin
- frequent urination/incontinence
- irregular periods/heavy bleeding
- feeling irritable
- vaginal dryness
- itchy skin
- loss of libido
- new facial hair
- anxiety
- headaches
- light-headed feeling
- weight gain
- heart palpitations.

Causes of perimenopause

What exactly causes our bodies to go into perimenopause?

When we are in our mid to late thirties, oestrogen and progesterone begin to decrease. It's a slow and natural process, so slow that we do not even notice, and this eventually leads us to perimenopause. As our ovaries, which produce oestrogen and progesterone, manufacture less and less, we begin to feel . . . different. Our bodies and our brain function may change; you may notice a distinct difference in your mood swings.

Oestrogen plays a great part in regulating mood-boosting properties. These include serotonin, norepinephrine and dopamine. The three feel-good buddies. These are super important for our state of mind and our sleep.

Oestrogen also affects our brain function, especially our cognition. Decreases in oestrogen can also cause some women to have occasional episodes of forgetfulness, or 'fuzzy-brain', which may lead to forgetting your PIN number at the checkout, your husband's birthday or that shiny thing you stir your tea with. (It's called a spoon, I remembered eventually.)

Of course, there are the physical changes that can also have an effect on your mood. Sleepless nights are a right pain the arse; trouble with sex, or rather, no sex at all, can not only cause anxiety and stress, but also challenges in your relationship.

Oestrogen and progesterone decrease, which causes your hormones to fluctuate, and this is what causes the change in your cycle. You may have found that you have extra-heavy bleeding or very irregular periods. Once your ovaries stop producing eggs you are in menopause.

In some women menopause is medically induced. Radiation and or pelvic injuries are the most common cause. An injury to the ovaries or surgical removal of the ovaries will bring about early menopause due to the fact that the ovaries are the main source of oestrogen production. Removal of the uterus, a hysterectomy, causes your periods to stop, but does not affect menopause as you still have your ovaries.

On a good note, surgical menopause can sometimes be a life-saver to women who have a history of ovarian and breast cancer in their families. The removal of the ovaries has also been known to sometimes assist with the pain of endometriosis.

Once you are postmenopausal, your hormones will not be fluctuating, they will remain at a low level. Hence no more periods, no more pregnancies.

Like so many other experiences in life, every woman's body is totally different. Just as giving birth can be extremely different from one woman to the next, so can menopause. There are many things you can do to help you through. We will visit those later in the book. I'm still experimenting with my symptoms. Some things work for a little while, then something in my body shifts and that lets me know I need to look for an alternative.

Younger self

I wonder, what did my younger self need to hear about menopause before coming to the age where I'd experience it myself?

I would have loved to have known what other women went through. What are the differing characteristics of menopause for women? How did they deal with the symptoms? What helped ease the symptoms? What was the outcome for them once they were out of perimenopause and fully in the swing of menopause? What happens at the end of it all?

Give me something to hang my hat on; give me something I can look forward to. Show me the light at the end of the tunnel.

I've been visiting quite a few alternative methods, which is my speed anyway, and I've also researched and read about many more modalities that can support you through menopause. I'm clearly not a doctor, therapist, naturopath or life coach. But if I can make you laugh a little, make you feel not so alone, and even sprinkle in some positivity for you, then I am happy. Very happy.

Don't trust people who don't laugh.

Maya Angelou
....

Menopause quiz

Q. Do goldfish really have a memory of three seconds?

A. If they are female and aged between 40 and 60, then yes.

Q. Which planets in our solar system are known as the gas giants?

A. Jupiter, Saturn, Uranus, Neptune and Planet Hormone.

Q. Can you lick your elbow?

A. If it means cooling myself off in a hot flush then *yes*, I will find a way.

Q. How many calories does sex burn?

A. Don't care, the walk to the fridge for chocolate will be more enjoyable at this point.

Q. Which mammal holds the record of having the shortest duration of sexual intercourse?

A. The chimpanzee, at an average of three seconds. Or a menopausal woman who could possibly do it in 2.89 seconds.

Q. What are 'entrance' and 'driveway' and 'menopause' in Swedish?

A. 'Infart' and 'utfart' and 'needtofart'.

Q. What is the highest ever recorded temperature on Earth?

A. A menopausal woman in summer.

Q. What is in a bed but never sleeps?

A. A perimenopausal woman.

Q. Which Tasmanian animal is known for its fiery temper?

A. Sheryl, she's 48 and six months into perimenopause.

Q. What's a four-letter word that ends in K and means the same as intercourse?

A. Talk.

Q. What does every woman have that starts with a 'V' and can be used to get what she wants?

A. Her voice.

Q. What sort of sexual practice is lectamia?

A. Caressing in bed without intercourse, also known as menopausal sex.

Q. What TV character must have sex every seven years?

A. Mr Spock . . . my dream guy.

Handle with care

How often as women have we passed off period cramps, menstrual headaches, dizzy spells and foggy brain as, 'It's just my period'.

The truth is, yes, of course it *is* your period, and the symptoms you might be experiencing due to perimenopause are *just* your hormones.

But wait.

We need to take all our symptoms seriously, handle them with care. Not just brush them off as they were so often brushed off in our youth when we were crumpled up in a heap from cramps and felt we had to somehow ignore them.

My youngest daughter called me from school the other day, in tears as she told me about the cramps she was having. She'd never experienced them before, or at least not to that extent. When I reached the school office she climbed into my arms and cried. Period cramps are no joke, and ask anyone with endometriosis about the pain that comes along with their cycle. The feeling of period cramps is unique. They can be painful. I remember as a young teenager rocking my body back and forth in an attempt to ease the cramping, feeling like the pain was never going to end.

The names we have given our cycle, like 'The Curse' or 'Female Trouble', don't exactly conjure an image of a wonderful, nurturing experience. And yet we continue on each month, often with the same cramping, sometimes even vomiting from the pain. We need to hold our daughters with more care in the same way we need to hold ourselves with care as we transition through perimenopause.

History

The history of menopause is nothing short of horrendous. We've made progress, thank heavens, though there's still more we can do to normalise menopause and take it out of the 'ailment' category and into the 'wellness' section.

The ancient Greeks (and I'm pretty damn sure it was a male who came up with this doozy) believed the uterus could sometimes become adrift inside a woman's body and jiggle around, resulting in unbridled emotion. The best remedy for this, they thought, was rigorous sex.

Aha, right.

Often the *last* thing a menopausal woman feels like having, this was clearly not a remedy any female concurred with.

Women are still dismissed as crazy or irrational because of 'that time of the month'.

In an article written by Jackie Rosenhek regarding menopause through the ages, she mentions the Salem trials, where sixteen women were accused of witchcraft. Thirteen of those targeted were over 50. This was a group of women thought to be powerful and threatening, and most likely they were . . . to the men in Salem.

She goes on to explain that the English physician Thomas Sydenham (1624–1689) noted that women between the ages of 45 and 50 were prone to 'hysterick fits' (had a few of those myself) and the only cure was to restore their cycle by blood-letting, a medieval form of doctoring that occurred by nicking a vein or artery and letting blood flow to balance the body. Like we needed more bleeding?

The French physician Charles Pierre Louis De Gardanne coined the term 'De la ménépausie', otherwise known as menopause, in 1821. From what I've read we can thank him for creating and spreading the first real negative attitudes towards this natural cycle in a woman's life.

The Victorian mindset hammered down the idea that menopause was a mental illness that needed to be cured. The doctors in England began prescribing douches containing lead (of all things), chloroform and morphine.

What followed were more male doctors thinking that the removal of the ovaries would fix everything. Even worse, a certain Dr Isaac Baker Brown (1811–1873) decided removing the clitoris, often without the woman's consent, in surgery would be a wonderful idea for 'fixing menopause'.

Women were institutionalised for menopause-induced hysteria and at one time it was believed that Jack the Ripper was a midwife and a menopausal woman.

I mean, COME ON.

Quack medicines and snake oils abounded to find a cure for menopause. Victorian pharmacies sold powdered ovaries and testicles—from where? I shudder to think. Most likely pig parts.

Nothing like ingesting testicles to fix menopause.

So, you see what we are up against?

This long line of history in the Western world has deemed us crazy, unstable and diseased in some way.

An article includes menopausal treatments from the 1800s and early 1900s that varied from the gruesome to the downright dangerous:

- mustard hip-baths (okay, relaxing in a bath, yes, I like it)
- *pediluvio* (also known as a foot bath—sure, love a nice foot soak)
- frictions with stimulating embrocations (basically a good massage, sign me up)
- electric therapy (yeah, nope)
- opium (nope)
- cold water directed to the abdomen (Why? Okay, maybe this would cool you down on a hot day)
- the filtered juice of guinea pigs' ovaries (What in the hell?)
- a vaginal plug and iced injections on its removal (Who came up with this one?)
- arsenic (poison, always a great remedy)
- thyroid gland extract (no thanks)
- golf (this made me laugh out loud—I had to wonder if somehow my husband had added this in here)
- orgasm (100%).[1]

My beginning

I was around the age of 45. I'd been dealing with changes in my body for a while. At first I joked about it, then I worried about all the things that might happen. Then it got real. The sweats, mood swings, weight gain, changes in my skin, my hair. My laundry list of vitamins and tonics skyrocketed.

I started exercising again after basically barely moving my body for twelve years when I 'accidentally' lost my fitness on the hospital floor after giving birth to my third child. Still, the weight gain, the aches, the joint issues. And along came perimenopause.

I could go on, write an epitaph about all the loss. But, like aging in general, I refuse to believe that it's all downhill. Aging is not a disease. There is change, yes. There is pain, hell yes. I do believe in the phoenix somewhere inside of me and she will rise. Even if she has to take more turmeric to do it.

Like death and taxes, menopause, if you are a woman, is on your life path, and if you are a partner to a woman, well, there's a possibility that sometimes we may need to apologise for what we've said, didn't say, threw at you, screamed at you and everything in between. I swear we didn't mean it . . . much.

My symptoms

I noted a change in my cycle. I'd always been regular, give or take a day or two, but then I noticed I'd have a cycle every two weeks, or I'd have a cycle that was so unbelievably heavy I could have been a shoe-in for a remake of *Carrie*.

Oh, and the belly grew, yes she did.

Let me put it this way: my 'nether regions' seemed to have disappeared under a fairly good-sized muffin top. I mean, I caught a glimpse if I heaved the belly upwards and sucked in, but generally that 'zone' was gone.

Look, I'm not blaming perimenopause entirely for my weight gain—there are other factors such as genetics, stress and lack of sleep. Mostly, though, I'd stopped exercising. And just in case no one ever mentions this . . . when you stop moving your body it causes weight gain.

There it is, in black and white. What a revelation, right?

I was a full-time preschool teacher, and my husband travelled constantly, so I had three kids to look after on my own. There was no time and certainly no energy for exercise. It was so far down my list of priorities to take care of my health through exercise—a fleeting thought. Add the hormonal shifts happening in my body and, well . . . the tummy, thighs and bum took on a life of their own. All three decided, 'Let's get this show on the road and *grow*, shall we, and let's invite that party animal cellulite along, too.'

The number of times I had to explain to people, 'No I'm not pregnant, just fat' was embarrassing. Convincing people that I really, truly was not six months along was ridiculous. I loved my pregnant belly and shape during all three of my pregnancies. But this looking pregnant without actually being pregnant was very unsatisfying.

Strangely, though, I had cravings like a pregnant woman, cravings for things I know I should not be eating, mostly sugar, red wine and potato chips (extra salty). Man, I craved them.

Who am I kidding? I still do.

I've since found out that both menopause and aging affect your metabolism. I used to be able to cut things out of my diet and exercise to maintain a healthy weight but, now, nothing was shifting.

No matter what I changed.

My energy level to actually do exercise was almost flatline, so the weight continued to blossom.

All this was happening while beginning to get ready to move from Los Angeles to Sydney. After 25 years of living in America.

I was visiting my naturopath at regular intervals to attempt to get some help with my exhaustion and food cravings and generally feeling unwell. What I learned was that I was in the midst of severe exhaustion, and that can go hand in hand with triggering King Kong–sized perimenopausal symptoms.

It's a bit like the chicken and the egg. If your body is taxed, it can mess with your hormones, and if your hormones are out of balance, you can feel more tired.

I was already an emotional wreck over leaving my friends and the place we had called home for a quarter of a century. So, between the beginning of perimenopause and my existing emotional state, I had was headed for a perfect storm of symptoms.

I stepped into the arena of perimenopause with nothing left in the tank. I had beautiful friends telling me I needed to take care of myself, and I had read self-help books about needing to look after 'me'. I understood the theory, though I never took action. It's one of those time-machine moments where I wish I could go back and tell myself to go a little easier.

I was not at my healthiest. With the lack of exercise and also a lack of sleep, my body was not happy. Though, like most of us women, I believed I just had to keep going. Other symptoms like brain fog, anxiety and mood swings I passed off as just my feelings around leaving America—I didn't connect them to perimenopause. Looking back, I was definitely going through a lot more, physically, than I realised. There was no time to rest and recuperate. Three kids, one dog, and a whole life to pack up, while riding everyone else's emotional rollercoasters, was one of the most draining experiences I've ever had.

Self-care

If I knew what I know now about the level of exhaustion I was at and how it plays a part in menopause, I would like to think I would have taken better care of myself.

So, if you are just at the beginning of perimenopause, or still in it, self-care needs to be at the top of your to-do list.

I say that like it's an easy thing to do. For me, it wasn't. Self-care? I didn't even know what that was half the time. Sometimes I thought online shopping could be considered 'self-care'. Apparently, it's not. Unfortunately, neither is falling asleep on the couch after overdosing on chocolate biscuits.

Self-care is elusive if you've never treated yourself to it. Especially if you're a mother, you work, or do both, or are a *woman* and were raised to put other people ahead of yourself.

Is self-care something you struggle with?

It's taken my deep plunge into health issues to understand how much self-care I need. And by this I mean care of your emotions and spirit, not just your physical self. Do not underestimate the importance of looking after you. I did, and I paid the price when perimenopause came a-knocking.

Start today. Actually, start yesterday. Please, if you are raising children, raise them with self-care. Demonstrate to them what a woman does to take care of herself, rather than how she sacrifices her own needs, feelings and health for others. As women we are up against an invisible ceiling that wants to keep us limited in terms of care and how much we can have, ask for, and demand. Sacrificing ourselves for others benefits no one.

You won't regret taking my advice.

Letter to my menopause

Dear Menopause,

Well, well, well, didn't you arrive in a rush, dressed in a red turtleneck jumper? Yes, my husband hates you, sorry, but he's learning about you as well. I'll invite you in, give you a long, tall glass of iced water. And I'll listen, I'll listen to everything you have to say. I know you have a lot to share, though sometimes, could you lower your voice? When you scream at me I retreat into myself and it's hard to take the wisdom. I need to get to know you better; I need to make friends, as I think you're here for a while. Let's agree to be gentle with each other, yeah? I'll hold your hand if you hold mine.

Love,
Me

CHAPTER 3

Hot stuff

Journal entry, February 2018

Armageddon. This is how I feel today. It's the heat, both internal and external. Feel like I'm cooking from the inside out. Feel like I'm going mad. Literally mad in this heat. What's the term . . . ? 'Going Troppo.' That's a real thing, I googled it. People losing their minds due to constant, inextinguishable heat.

Also, what's with the conspiracy theories running through my brain lately? And the panic about my children and the million ways they could be killed? What's this fresh delight? Lately the 3 a.m. wakeups have been smothered with a feeling of worry. So much so that I'm finding myself launching from the bed, alert to something that I feel has gone wrong, or some kind of danger. Thoughts of watching my children being eaten alive by a crocodile run through my head, amping up the adrenaline so the chance of sleep becomes non-existent. A crocodile? For the love of God, I live in Sydney—chances that death by crocodile will happen are as likely as me growing a third leg.

Which may or may not also be a nightmare of mine.

Fever, in the morning, fever all through the night . . .

I think of all the things perimenopause signals, the most common is the hot flushes. Hot flushes are strange.

It's not like when you are running a fever; it's a different kind of heat.

Before I hit perimenopause, I watched other women reach for a fan or a piece of paper to get some relief from the heat. My girlfriends stripping off layers as the hot flush lit them up from the inside.

I didn't understand what they were really feeling.

Well, I do now! For me it's a tingly all over, head-about-to-explode feeling. It's as if someone has shot me full of adrenaline and turned the heat to extreme. They are so random as well, for seemingly no rhyme or reason, at rest or out and about, I suddenly find myself engulfed in sweat.

Night-time is a different beast.

And what a beast it is . . . The hurl of the bedclothes across the bed, the windows can't be open enough, and getting back to sleep can take hours.

When I wake up at (as I've heard it called) 'dark thirty', it's like there's a disco happening in my brain and DJ Uterus has been playing the same song on repeat all night. I will have not only the song, but random thoughts about my day, lists of things I need to do, and another voice attempting to tell someone (I don't know who) to 'TURN THE MUSIC DOWN'. All the while, there's another voice telling me to take deep breaths.

My mum calls the music a 'brain worm'.

I've also heard that the song you simply cannot boot from your brain has a message for you in the lyrics.

Interesting.

My last go round with a song has been 'Youngblood' by 5 Seconds of Summer. The song lyrics the eager young singer states are he's 'like a dead man walking'.

Isn't *that* an ironic message for a menopausal woman? I don't think it takes Freud to figure it out.

Yes, my 'youngblood' has left the premises. And have I felt like a 'dead man walking'? Sure, at times.

Menopause playlist

'Ring of Fire'—Johnny Cash

'Burning Down the House'—Talking Heads

'Set Fire to the Rain'—Adele

'I'm on Fire'—Bruce Springsteen

'Just Like Fire'—Pink

'Girl on Fire'—Alicia Keys

'Beds Are Burning'—Midnight Oil

'Burning Love'—Elvis Presley

'Burning up'—Madonna

'Fire Down Below'—Tina Turner

'Soul on Fire'—Kylie Minogue

'The Heat Is On'—Glenn Frey

'My Heat Goes Boom'—Snoop Dogg

'Cold Sweat'—Thin Lizzy

'Hot N Cold'—Katy Perry

Power surges

So, what to do with these night-time volcanic moments?

I've needed to learn how to either get myself back to sleep or use the time for myself.

At first when the wakeups/hot flushes began—along with the annoying songs, the swirling thoughts, worries, and sweat cascading from my body and sticking me to the sheets—I didn't know what to do. I would toss and turn, getting more panicked as the clock ticked over another hour, knowing I needed to be up and functioning soon.

Some nights I would cry because I couldn't find any way back to sleep.

When the sun did rise, I would finally drag myself from the bed. I was not only exhausted but grouchy as hell.

I have noticed that red wine tends to beckon these nights a little more, hence my pulling back on drinking. I do miss it a little. But not being a big drinker in the first place, I shifted my view to how it's *good* for me to be off alcohol, and I remind myself it's not forever.

I've also been checking out certain foods, what fulfills me, what bloats, what keeps me up at night.

Have you noticed anything in your diet that worsens symptoms of perimenopause? For me it's all the usual bad guys: sugar, wheat, caffeine and fried foods.

I will own up: I did not give up my black tea. Nothing, no one, no how, will get between me and my tea. It's in my blood, it's my meditation, my relaxation. I just shifted my last cup to a bit earlier so the caffeine would not interfere with my sleep.

Who am I kidding? What is sleep anyway? I mean, *everything* seems to interfere with sleep, right?

Leaving tea completely out of my diet is a step too far; I will most likely be found dead in my chair at a ripe old age with a cup of tea grasped in my arthritic hands.

Tea brings me joy.

I'm giving sage tea a go before bed at night and taking my menopause pills religiously. Drinking more water throughout the day helps. The internal heat causes me to feel somewhat dehydrated. Dehydration = headaches. Hormonal shifts also cause headaches; you might have experienced this with your period. Perimenopause can bring similar symptoms as PMS. So keep the water levels high.

Changing my diet has helped. Where I was willing to overlook how certain foods reacted in my body before perimenopause, I'm now not willing to eat the crap food, feel terrible *and* have menopausal symptoms.

I can't control perimenopause arriving at my doorstep with her array of symptoms. But I can control what I eat, so I made a start trying to cut things out.

I need to remind myself sometimes to actually *thank* menopause. I am most definitely healthier than I've been in years.

Daytime hot flushes are way more manageable than the night-time ones. In the daytime I can easily cope and simply cool myself down by taking a walk outside, ripping all my clothes off and burying myself in the snow.

I wish.

I live in Sydney, where we have no snow, damnit. Though I have been known to open the freezer door and stick my head in for a bit. There have been winter nights when the heater has been on, and my family sit at the dinner table in their jumpers, and I sit in shorts and a bra and my face flame red.

Too dang hot for clothes.

To help me fall back to sleep now, I use my breath. I imagine my breath filling me up from my toes to my head and then out again from head to toe. I also tell myself, 'Be here now'. A request for my brain to stop running ahead into the future worrying about crap I have absolutely no control over in the dark of my bedroom at 3.37 in the morning.

I write a list of things I need to do for the following day so it's not rattling around my brain. I make sure my bedroom is tidy—something about a messy room makes me not sleep well. Absolutely no TV/phone screens in the bedroom.

Some dim lighting. And a great book helps also.

If all else fails, and I can't lie there for a second longer, the dark thirty wakeups have me reading more, writing more, or having some seriously nice quiet time.

You see, that way you can use your sleepless nights due to hot flushes as a power surge.

Knowing that the hot flush will eventually settle down helps me to remember that 'this too shall pass'.

Having a plan of something lovely to do for yourself when the heat hits transforms these flushes from little bits of hell to little bits of heaven.

What can you plan out for your 3 a.m. rendezvous with a hot flush?

If sleep isn't happening, then see if you can find an enjoyable way to pass the time. Do something that eases your mind and keeps you relaxed, if possible.

Journal entry, April 2018

Here you come again. The swirl. The pull of defeat and judgement. What am I doing with my life? I have no purpose. I have no talent, no direction. Why am I writing this book? I'm so stupid. No one cares. My body hurts; my knees, hips, back. I'm tired from the heat I feel. Every night I'm woken by hot flushes: push the covers off, feel chilly, pull the covers up— repeat, all night. The sleeplessness has begun again, day after day, wearing down my resilience, my patience, my ability to lift myself up from the fog of nothingness. I'm turning in circles, looking for my way out. But all I want to do is sleep. Lie down.

Is that okay? Can I give myself over to the fog? I'm nervous, scared as to how far I'll be lost in it. I like the quiet. Don't want to be around anyone. I want peace. Don't pull at me; errands and boring shit don't interest me. Family coming today. I don't want to pretend that I'm all 'up' and 'good'. I'd like to just sit ever so quietly—breathe, read, sleep. That's it. What if I tip? The edge of the cliff looks nearer today. Not to jump, just to warn me—don't fall into the abyss. If only I could rest my brain at night. Just to feel the release of a good night's sleep would balance me, help me. The crease between my brow grows ever deeper. I frown in my sleep when I don't sleep deeply. My brain tossing around every thought from the meaning of life to what I can make for lunch today. Need sleep, that blank, soft, kind sleep. Rejuvenating sleep. Too much Instagram, reading other people's lives; being sucked into the void of external interest never works for me. Deadens my soul, my creativity. Need to find something in my life to live for. Something that excites me and gets me out of bed with a spring in my step. Babies used to do that, toddlers used to do that. I feel so lazy. My arms feel like lead. I've got to change this.

Letter to my uterus

Dear Uterus,

Congratulations! Early retirement for you, my friend. You did a mighty fine job, you carried three beautiful humans incredibly well. You contracted when you were meant to each month.

Are you tired? Would you like a rest, retire from cramping and pushing? Let me say thank you, I love you; you gave me the best dream-fulfilling presents ever. Kick back. Stay healthy and hydrated.

Love,
Me

CHAPTER 4

Shame, vulnerability and anger, oh my

Emotions make us human, denying them makes us beasts.

VICTORIA KLEIN

Dr Mary Jane Minkin, a professor in obstetrics, gynaecology, and reproductive health at Yale Medical School and lead author of a study on the cultural impact of menopause, writes:

> In societies where age is more revered and the older woman is the wiser and better woman, menopausal symptoms are significantly less bothersome. Where older is not better, many women equate menopause with old age, and symptoms can be much more devastating.[1]

Every single woman will go through menopause. Whether it be naturally or through necessary surgery. That's an amazing statistic, don't you think? Again, it blows my mind that programmed into our bodies is future menopause. It cannot be undone, denied, avoided. All those Kardashian women—menopause. All those Victoria's Secret girls—menopause. Anyone you may have compared yourself to, felt less than as you watched Instagram posts of her youthful body, yep—menopause. It's coming for those ladies, too.

We can get ready for it. I want you to get ready for it. I wish I had.

I truly believe we can/must *have all our feelings* around this topic, and this extends to many things: aging in general, body image, fertility, expectations of women, career change, marriage/divorce/relationship breakdown, depression, anxiety.

I intend to keep doing exactly that.

HAVING. ALL. MY. FEELINGS.

As you are shifting, you will begin to realise that you are not the same person you used to be. The things you used to tolerate have now become intolerable. Where you once remained quiet, you are now speaking your truth. Where you once battled and argued, you are now choosing to remain silent. You are beginning to understand the value of your voice, and there are some situations that no longer deserve your time, energy or focus.

@mich_hyde
....

Vulnerability

Menopause has brought me to my knees in terms of vulnerability. I tell myself it's okay to be and feel vulnerable. Even when I'm running—okay, maybe not running, because of my dodgy knees, but a super quick power walk—in the opposite direction, and lying to everyone along the way— 'I'm fine', 'all good here', 'no problems'—in fact, I'm not fine, I'm not all good, and I feel like I have a million problems.

I've felt the most vulnerable around my husband and being physically intimate. Letting him know that there were changes happening in my body that made the experience of intimacy uncomfortable. That I was afraid he saw me as ugly, because I saw myself as ugly. I felt vulnerable when I didn't want to get out of bed some days and I could not stop crying at things that didn't make sense to me. When I realised that my baby-making years were gone.

When I do actually allow myself to be vulnerable, to be honest, to lie down belly up and ask for help, and share my fears, I inevitably feel so much better. I love vulnerability in other people and I've learned to love it in myself. I feel the softness that comes with it. I feel the aftermath of being exposed and truthful and having survived being honest about how I feel.

Shame

Of all the emotions I feel, the one I am most troubled by is shame. Shame around not being good enough, smart enough, around thinking I was more 'evolved', or simply a better person. I describe it as a living, breathing doorway to hell. How do I come to terms with all the changes within my body and emotions?

But why *shame* when it comes to the changes in my physicality?

Why has my worth been so tied up with how I look? Should my size and whether or not I have love handles affect how much shame I have about myself? I've somehow felt responsible for keeping a youthful image not only for myself but for others around me, as though I have done something wrong by simply aging. It has pained me to feel this way, knowing that the message I've been telling myself is the worst kind of example to set for my daughters, let alone any other woman I might come into contact with. This view of what's important sounds vain. But I know, in resisting it, I am attempting to uproot so many generational and societal beliefs alongside my own.

I hate shame. Nothing positive or kind comes from shaming anyone, no lessons are learned, and no motivation is ignited. Shame is a crushed underfoot, belittling emotion. It makes me believe that I am unlovable by simply being me.

> I define shame as the intensely painful feeling or experience of believing that we are flawed and therefore unworthy of love and belonging—something we've experienced, done, or failed to do makes us unworthy of connection. I don't believe shame is helpful or productive.[2]
>
> *Brené Brown*
> ....

You might have heard of Dr Brené Brown, a research professor at the University of Houston's Graduate School of Social Work who has studied topics such as shame, vulnerability and worthiness. I pretty much hang off every word this woman speaks or writes. I have found her to be so refreshingly honest yet so informative around tough subjects like shame. Her TED Talk on vulnerability is one of the most downloaded TED Talks of all time. If you've seen it, you'll know why. Genius. Brené has been a strong proponent of sharing your vulnerability—essentially, admitting your feelings of shame so you can be more connected to others. She says:

Shame cannot survive being spoken and met with empathy. What it craves is secrecy, silence and judgement. If you stay quiet, you stay in self-judgement.

Shame for women is this web of unattainable, conflicting, competing expectations about who we are supposed to be . . . and it's a straitjacket.

There it is: 'who we are *supposed* to be'. According to whom? What shape am I *supposed* to be? What lines and bumps am I not *supposed* to have?

Dang, it's like gum on my shoes attempting to shake this ever-present ideal of what women should be/look like. And I've bought into it hook, line and sinker. Starting out as a model set me up for heavy expectations on aging. There is a lot more to unpack here for me for sure.

Empathy and kindness towards myself, speaking my shame out loud and to the right person help, a lot. It's another aspect of the wild ride that is menopause. Uprooting the origin of the belief systems that were planted in me from a young age.

Perfectionism is a self-destructive and addictive belief system that fuels this primary thought: if I look perfect, and do everything perfectly, I can avoid or minimise the painful feelings of shame, judgement and blame.

Brené Brown
....

Anger

The older I get, the more I see how women are described as having gone mad, when what they've become is knowledgeable and powerful and fucking furious.

Sophie Heawood
....

I mention anger many times in this book—how I've felt rageful and angry at small things. Things that don't deserve my righteous anger.

I am working to shift the anger that surges out of nowhere, like a hidden beast that wants to scratch and claw at someone to get relief, by adding humour when possible, exiting the room or taking a deep breath.

Though the anger that I am loving, that I am wrapping my arms around, is this bright clear, red-hot belly anger. Anger at all the things I never spoke up about, anger at things that are unjust, unkind, cruel.

Anger when wielded correctly is a powerful, mountain-moving emotion, and I'm really beginning to love mine.

Anger protects me and the ones I love. Anger is the source from which I draw compassion when something is unfair. Anger enables me to take action to change what's wrong, and for me to align myself with my heart and desires.

I just finished reading a biography of Stevie Nicks, the little blonde powerhouse lead singer from Fleetwood Mac. Stevie went through the ultimate lifestyle of sex, drugs (so much drugs), fights, abortions, rehab, weight gain, antidepressants, addiction. She lived the total 1970s rockstar chick's life. When Stevie was going through menopause, she wanted to talk about it to the press—she had always been open with her life and her mental health struggles. Her agents and managers all said, 'No, it will ruin your career!' Here's what's amazing, after all that she'd lived through, they wanted her to hide the fact she was in menopause. Seriously? Sure, share the fact you snorted mounds of cocaine up your nose every week, but God forbid you mention you are having hot flushes. How insulting. I guess they thought menopause and rock chick don't align. And yes, she was rightfully *angry* that something as natural as menopause was to be kept secret in order for her image to not to be ruined. Ridiculous.

And women, I encourage you to acknowledge your fury.
Give it language. Share it in safe places of identification
and in safe ways. Your fury is not something to be afraid of.
It holds lifetimes of wisdom. Let it breathe and listen.[3]

Tracee Ellis Ross
....

Soraya Chemaly

Soraya Chemaly is a feminist writer, critic and activist whose work focuses on women's rights and the role of gender in politics, religion and popular culture.

Her entire TED Talk on anger and women hits the nail right on the head when she says, 'In culture after culture, anger is reserved as the moral property of boys and men. And so we teach children to disdain anger in girls and women, and we grow up to be adults that penalise it.'

She goes on to ask the question, 'So what if we didn't do that? What if we didn't sever anger from femininity?'

I love her response.

Because severing anger from femininity means we sever girls and women from the emotion that best protects us from injustice.

In the same way that we learned to cross our legs and tame our hair, we learned to bite our tongues and swallow our pride.

Furthermore, she explains the difference between how women and men are able to express their anger:

In anger, we go from being spoiled princesses and hormonal teens, to high-maintenance women and shrill, ugly nags. Whether we're at home or in school or at work or in a political arena, anger confirms masculinity, and it confounds femininity. So, men are rewarded for displaying it, and women are penalised for doing the same.

I mentioned earlier in the book my struggle with being the 'nice girl' and a 'people pleaser'. This is a common one among women. Soraya goes on to say how women are at a disadvantage with our anger, especially if we need to defend ourselves and our own interests: 'If we're faced with a threatening street harasser, predatory employer, a sexist, racist classmate, our brains are screaming, "Are you kidding me?" And our mouths say, "I'm sorry, what?"'

If men knew how often women were filled with white hot rage when we cried, they would be staggered.

We use minimising language. 'I'm frustrated. No, really, it's okay.'

My experience of sexual assault makes me think about how I was not trained to be stronger, to know my boundaries, afraid that I would offend my attacker if I clearly stated that he should leave at the doorway. I say this with no judgement against myself, but an understanding of how women's anger needs a beautiful, clear voice.

I am a big believer in the body–mind connection. Our thoughts create our reality and can directly affect our health. I know this to be true from my own experiences with my health and wellness. Soraya explains anger and the body like this:

We self-objectify and lose the ability to even recognise the physiological changes that indicate anger. Mainly, though, we get sick. Anger has now been implicated in a whole array of illnesses that are casually dismissed as 'women's illnesses'. Higher rates of chronic pain, autoimmune disorders, disordered eating, mental distress, anxiety, self-harm, depression. Anger affects our immune systems, our cardiovascular systems.

I am sick and tired of the women I know being sick and tired. Our anger brings great discomfort, and the conflict comes because it's our role to bring comfort. There is anger that's acceptable. We can be angry when we stay in our lanes and buttress the status quo. As mothers or teachers, we can be mad, but we can't be angry about the tremendous costs of nurturing. We can be angry at other women, because who doesn't love a good catfight?

People who are able to process their anger and make meaning from it are more creative, more optimistic, they have more intimacy, they're better problem solvers, they have greater political efficacy.

One thing that has driven me nuts is when other people attempt to downplay *my* feelings, with a well-meaning, 'You'll be fine' or, 'Whatever, get over it'. When I am sharing how I'm feeling, especially in the depths of my sadness that has felt so confusing to me, to be wiped away with a dismissive comment is more than not helpful, it's hurtful. The same can be said as to how I speak to myself. While there is a fine line between wallowing in self-pity and allowing myself to have all my feelings, the worst thing I could possibly do is ignore or belittle how I'm feeling.

Yes, we may want to be 'over it', though without really feeling what's happening and understanding as best we can what the hell is going on with us, we might experience a build-up of emotions that are bound to either come out sideways in a rush towards someone we love (usually) or turn inwards, where we punish ourselves for not 'feeling happy'. Both of these scenarios are devastating.

As you grow and evolve you might feel like you're losing your mind. But you are losing your old mindset that was holding you back.

@herincrediblemindset
....

Depression or mood swing?

Writing in a journal has been something I've done since I was in my twenties. It's assisted me with an incredible amount of brain chatter and thoughts that need to be purged from my mind. Seeing my thoughts down on paper helps me enormously. My 3.30 a.m. wakeups have not always been fun—far from it. Yet I've used that quiet time to write in my journal. I do still wrestle with the turning over and over of events, and especially self-doubt. Things I did or didn't say. I run the questioning gauntlet between, 'Do I wax my legs Tuesday or Thursday?' To 'What am I doing with my life?'

June of 2018 was an especially dark time for me. There were no real triggers, just a steady decline into a deep sadness that had me barely able to get out of bed. At times I felt terrified of how far down the well of despair I'd fallen. I like to think that I'm usually an optimist, though with the hormonal rollercoaster I was on, not even my happy place—my children—could help me see the sunshine.

Journal entry, June 2018

Wept today,
Wept for my body that no longer gives life,
Wept for my friendships that no longer surround me,
Wept for my happiness that seems to elude me,
Wept for a life that is shattered and meaningless,
Wept for my light that has been extinguished,
Wept for my children born and unborn,
Wept for the mother I was and never will be again,
Wept for the advice that dried in my mouth to my daughters.

What slippery slope am I on? I don't understand my life right now. It's like everything I've been keeping at bay has caught up with me: age, wrinkles, fat—God, I'm so fat can't believe how my body looks. I don't feel like me. My face is so ugly, too. So droopy and sad and angry all at the same time. I dress myself up in the morning and I look like mutton dressed as lamb. So gross. My hair is a nightmare; it's gone so dry and weird. Something I used to rely on to look good now doesn't look good at all. Basically I've totally lost my looks. I see photos and barely recognise myself. I don't understand what's happened to me. Is it that all the shitty negative things in my brain have made their way to the external part of myself? My eyes are fucked—no eyelashes, so that looks hideous. There is nothing left of the beauty of my youth. Is this what menopause does? It's a cruel bitch if it does. Can't wear the clothes I want anymore: anything that's tight around the middle looks ridiculous, jeans look dumb, all my beautiful dresses are looking crap, too, because they look like maternity dresses now. I feel so sad and so lost. I'm standing in this forest alone growing old and feeling like I have no one who cares, no one who wants to know me, be around me. I have nothing interesting to share or give, no one wants my opinion on anything. Oh, to be asked, 'What do you think, or feel, about this?' Cam will continue to get fitter and fitter. That's great, though I feel so left behind. Can't keep up physically with anything. It's so frustrating. We go for a bike ride, and my family is always saying, 'Wait for Mum.' A hike: 'Wait for Mum.' Fuck. I can't stand it and I don't know what I'm meant to do. Rally? Take more action, think positive, chant, meditate? I don't want to help myself. That's the problem. The depression wants to take me under so badly it's all I can do to not let it drown me. It pulls at me to stay in bed, to not move, not reach out; to stay in my pyjamas all day while *it tells me I'm worthless, ugly, dumb. I bounce around from doctor to doctor trying to get some help. I get some help and the darkness pulls me right under again. I feel so full of hatred for myself. I can't remember ever feeling so ugly and crappy, so old and bitter, and it shows in my face. My face used to show the kindness and compassion I felt and now all I see is the judging eyes, the bitter mouth, the sad long droopy face. What am I meant to do? I feel like I should walk away, run away, go somewhere on my own, like Ireland, and live in a tiny cottage and breathe. Neck is hurting again. The disc is beginning to bulge. Great, yet another physical thing I've got to deal with. Don't talk about it. I see* Cam *roll his eyes when I have another ailment. So boring, so ugly, not fun, not interesting, and so dumb. So old and UGLY UGLY UGLY. Need help. Really, really need help. But what? How?*

The real difficulty is to overcome how you think about yourself.

Maya Angelou
....

Seeing the light

I take a long deep breath when I read that passage now. I love that Maya Angelou quote. It's so true—the difficulty I need to overcome is not so much menopause, it's how I think about myself.

Menopause just turns my feelings up to eleven.

That winter was the bleakest of winters for me. I've never considered myself to be a depressed person, though the state of mind I was in was the lowest I can ever remember feeling. I was in a very dark spin. I felt incredibly isolated. I felt my marriage was practically over. There was so much I didn't like about Cam that I couldn't feel anything loving towards him. Every word and action of his were like nails down a chalkboard.

Nothing prepared me for the feeling of simply, 'I don't care'. Those three words had never been extended to my children. But for the first time, that's how I felt. My three most treasured beings and I didn't care? I was horrified. But I so deeply and utterly didn't care about myself. That's when my junk food habit kicked way up. Staring endlessly at Instagram, isolating myself from my family and friends in Los Angeles and Australia, I was not engaging with anyone. And what terrified me the most was this loop of thought: 'Your family would be better off without you.' I started to believe that. I was too sad, too boring, too annoying, no fun, had nothing to offer. Worthless.

Sleep was of course a patchwork of small naps, which as you all know is the worst way to try to get a handle on anything. They don't use sleep deprivation as a form of torture in war for laughs. All the things that normally helped me with challenging situations felt a million miles away. I also had the attitude of, why bother, nothing *would* help anyway.

There was another part of me standing outside myself looking in and thinking, 'Where are you going with this? This is not you. You don't think like this.' But the thoughts kept at me. Lurking on the periphery of my brain. I would wake up hoping I'd reset myself, only to find the darkness was still in bed with me.

I attempted to just 'cheer up', to 'get over it'. All those bloody stupid catchphrases that never work when you are so far down the rabbit hole you can't see your own hand or anyone else reaching out to you. I felt sick. Mentally sick. I would sit in the shower and cry. I wore the sadness on my face like a mask.

I slowly saw the light again by talking more, seeing my beautiful naturopath who helped with not only my physical symptoms but my emotional ones, too. I spent more time outdoors, walking and listening to uplifting podcasts. Cam and I took a weekend away on a road trip. I asked for hugs. I watched funny movies. I started saying 'yes' to invites from new friends. Little steps that eased the darkness I felt.

Many months later, that time is now just a memory. I felt for a long time afterwards that depression was still waiting for me. That I would feel that way again. Like a physical injury that would flare from time to time with the wrong exercise. To this day, I've never slid so far down into the pit of despair as I did then. I've teetered on the edge a fair bit. I can't say exactly how I fell to the bottom of the pit, but I have some ideas. Was it mostly hormonal levels going crazy or a combination of things?

I don't believe perimenopause 'made me' depressed. I just know that from where I started, with such a lack of self-care and losing my support system, and then with those fluctuating hormones having their way with my body and brain, the only lens I could see the world through was negative.

There have been times in my life when I wasn't sure if I could keep going.

And there have been days when I have felt I couldn't deal with yet another day of perimenopause—I can't have another day of hot flushes, of not sleeping, of feeling like total crap. Yet how many times have we said that in our lives and survived another day, survived another hour, another week, month, year? We've survived when people we know and love have passed away, when our hearts have been broken, when we gave birth, raised a screaming toddler, had a horrific accident. All those times that we said to ourselves and others, 'I can't do this, I can't get through this,' we *did*. And you can.

Sometimes I still need to say, 'I feel like I can't do this menopause'—to hear that out loud. Because I know I've said those words about plenty of other moments in my life and yet here I am on the other side.

In the end, we will get through menopause. Because that's what we do. As women we are especially resilient creatures.

I think about my first pregnancy. I was in labour for 56 hours. When I'd hit the 47th hour I looked up at my doula and said, 'Can I do this?' She looked at me with a smile and said, 'Yes, you can, you *are* doing it.' So, to any of you who are struggling like me, who are feeling the physical and emotional pain of menopause, feeling like you can't do this, I'm here to tell you, *Yes you can*.

Remember, we've conquered harder things than menopause.

I'm at the age where my brain went from 'you probably shouldn't say that' to 'what the hell, let's see what happens'.

@rebelcircus

....

—

I've talked to so many women about their symptoms around perimenopause. One described herself as angry. So angry all the time. Another said she thought multiple times about driving her car into a tree at high speed.

In researching this particular element of perimenopause I find it's extremely alarming the number of women who feel suicidal.

Another woman mentioned she didn't feel suicidal from the symptoms, but from how her husband was treating her since starting perimenopause—because she no longer wanted sex, as it had become painful. She was juggling weight gain and other changes, and he berated her to the point she felt she could not take the bullying any longer.

These experiences can leave us feeling isolated. All the more reason to begin talking, sharing our menopause experiences as a common thread that links us all as women.

Our moods can be affected by many things, from an issue at work, to an argument with a family member. Sometimes it's not clear what causes mood swings and the irritability that often tailgates them. Mood swings also differ from depression. The good news is that clinical depression is not typically linked with menopause.

Clinical depression is a serious condition defined by intense sadness or despair that lasts more than two weeks, and that interferes with your daily life. It's possible to not realise the symptoms for a long time before you wake up and understand your life has become joyless. Looking back, I wouldn't have defined myself as clinically depressed; I had not experienced those feelings to that depth before, and haven't since. I guess what I had was an episode of depression. It was frightening and my heart goes out to anyone who deals with depression on a daily basis. Please, seek help if you feel this way.

New sense

On the flip side, the benefit—yes that's right, I said it, the *benefit*—of all this shifting and changing is that I have a new, emerging sense about my life.

I am done with coming in second, third or last place.

I feel like I'm waking up to a new sense of myself. And I like it.

One aspect about getting older I hear about over and over from women is this wonderful new attitude of not giving a crap. This has begun to take shape for me, too. Yes, I care just as much for the people and things that I love, but I don't overthink the small or petty crap—people not liking me, spending all day in my pyjamas, or saying what I want to say when I want to say it. Turning down anything I simply don't want to do. Of course, my people pleaser flares up every now and again, but generally I'm grateful I've joined the Don't Give a Crap Club.

Talking to women who are post menopausal, there is a common through line: a sense of strength in themselves, and not needing to please everyone else.

There is such a profound feeling related to making it to the midpoint in your life and feeling that you are about to start all over again—that you have a different outlook and an inner strength and wisdom that will guide you for the next half.

As females, it is instilled in us from an early age to simultaneously handle so many parts of our lives: work, children, partners, aging parents, etc. Women are the caregivers, though we often forget to care about ourselves.

Make saying 'no' a part of who you are, and say 'yes' to what nourishes your soul.

This is my favourite part about menopause. This is the freedom and the joy that can replace any sadness and loss.

Intuition/creativity

Hormonal imbalances that are a part of PMS, perimenopause and menopause exaggerate what's already there. I remember often around the time right before my cycle was due to begin I'd feel deeply connected to my intuition and my creativity. I found with PMS that while I was sensitive and a little snappier than usual, I was also aware of my feelings and those of the people around me so much more, and I was filled with ideas for things I wanted to do and make. I would take advantage of those times to either write an article or start an art project. My intuition at that time was usually pretty spot on, if I do say so myself. Everything felt heightened.

I've found perimenopause can be like PMS 24/7. I have this creative urge moving through me. I feel my sensitivity to people and feelings has been fine-tuned. This excites me. I have heard of many women who have found hidden creative talents later in life. As they have moved past the full-time mother/worker role and found time for themselves, their creativity has burst forth. Pretty exciting stuff. I just need to ride the wave of the highs and lows better so I'm not either clawing like a scared cat or creating masterpieces at the kitchen table at 3.30 a.m. A bit of balance, please.

How have the highs and lows been for you? Did you find you were more creative, connected to your feelings around your cycle? Have you noticed a shift in your creativity since becoming perimenopausal?

Starting over

If I look at menopause as a reset, as a new beginning, it's where I'm presented with the choice to choose myself. It's a beautiful moment. It can be a whole lot of beautiful moments strung together to make a new story for yourself. Where you are the lead character. Where you are the hero who rides in on the white horse, scooping up your sad and broken self and kissing her worried brow, her stretch marks, her tears.

I've so often waited for others to come and rescue me from my own emotions and feelings. What I know is that, at the end of the day, it's been me, and continues to be me, who picks myself up and dusts myself off again and again.

That's part of the deep sense of feeling alone in this change: it's all me, and it's all you, too. Partners, children or books are not going to assist me to feel any better unless I open myself up and truly allow them to.

It's been work and continues to be work for me to change my attitude about my menopause and my ever-changing body and mind. Consciously taking steps, no matter how small, towards being okay with all of my symptoms.

So maybe you and I are not Miss Menopause 2022 and have it all figured out. Just the fact that we are on the road to finding our way through this with laughter and love as companions is enough. And remember, there are a lot of women on the same road as us. We are hot and sweaty, some of us are out of shape, some of us will be yelling and swearing, and some may go skipping merrily along. But this path has been well worn, and it's far more enjoyable when we chat along the way.

Women's bodies, women's wisdom

Dr Christiane Northrup is one of the world's foremost authorities on women's health and wellness, teaching women how to thrive at every stage of life. I recommend her book *Women's Bodies, Women's Wisdom* as a treat for yourself. I have a well-worn copy and I often give the book as a gift. She is a leader in all things women, both physically and emotionally and especially how the two interact with each other. How we think about our bodies impacts how our bodies flourish or not.

She also has a website that she continues to update with relevant information. Especially pertaining to women and menopause.

In one particularly interesting article she explains how the patriarchal society and programming have a lot to do with how we think and care for our bodies. She writes that this has been part of our programming for over 5000 years and that it's 'no surprise that women get sick in the uniquely female areas of our bodies'.

Referencing the bible story of Adam and Eve, Dr Northrup describes it as 'the original sin of being born female', using the words of Anne Wilson Schaef. God banished Adam and Eve from the Garden of Eden and declared that Eve would bring forth children in pain and suffering, because she tempted Adam! Not for a moment do I think Eve was a hussy; back in the day Adam didn't have many other women to choose from, right? And I'm pretty darn sure Adam had some say in getting it on with Eve. This foundational language that defines at the core who we are as women also teaches us that the processes of the female body—menstrual cycles, pregnancy and menopause—are a burden to endure.

Add to that years of our culture telling us we are the wrong shape, size, colour, that we should wear makeup, not wear makeup, cinch our waists, let it all out, smile, look pretty, and that our bodies are simply not good enough.

Dr Northrup, continues, telling us, 'Our processes are embodied with wisdom and that whenever we trivialise our bodies or are ashamed of their normal processes, we are not only missing the clues, we are contributing to our own ill health.'

To control our bodies is to think in the terms of the patriarchy. I love it when she mentions how 'Our bodies work best when we love them the way we would a two-year-old child'. Something about that imagery just softens my heart to my body and my judgements. Never would I judge a two-year-old and be unkind. Being calm, kind and patient with myself is how I want to always be.[4]

Tips for falling in love with you

Mirror, mirror on the wall, who's the cutest of them all?

1. Cut the negative talk. I know, easier said than done. I still look at myself some days and lament about some part of me that I find ugly. This is not helpful. Finding just one thing you like about yourself and focusing on that alone can help shut down all the crappy negative talk. Compliment yourself as you would your best friend.

2. Gratitude is a cure-all for so many negative feelings. There have been times when I've looked at my legs and thought, 'Hello you beastly, dimply dragon legs. How the hell am I going to love you?' But these legs of mine, they work—a little rusty at times, sure, but they get me around just fine, so for that, I'm grateful. I still have all my bits and pieces and generally I'm in good health, and that alone gives me an enormous sense of gratitude.

3. Forgive yourself. This is a big one. I am so much harder on myself than anyone else in my life, but continuing to punish myself for saying or doing the wrong thing never helps. I have to forgive myself for all the things I didn't achieve or

finish. Hanging on to past mistakes keeps me trapped in the guilt.

4. Let go of the idea of being perfect. What even *is* perfect? I have driven myself crazy with comparisons to what other women are wearing, doing, saying, being. From thinking I've not given my kids the best school lunch, to comparisons for the best 'beach body'. I'm exhausted from attempting to be perfect. I'm *so* over 'perfect'. Because, really, perfect is simply being 100 per cent me.

5. Do something wonderful just for you. We are constantly told this, in women's magazines, from self-help gurus and in parenting tips. To make time for ourselves. I've found my desire to want to do more for myself has grown as I've aged, and I'm grateful for that. The idea that sacrifice is the normal way for women to operate is no longer valid to me.

Letter to my emotions

Dear Emotions,

Why are you all so loud? And wanting my attention constantly? And would all of you mind just relaxing, say, every second day? Take a break, you know? Just cruise in neutral for the day. Kick back. But most of all, please, oh please, go to sleep at night. As in, *all of you*, especially Mr Worry and Miss Negative—you both really need to shut the hell up.

Love,

Me

She has been feeling it for a while—that sense of awakening. There is a gentle rage simmering inside her, and it's getting stronger by the day. She will hold it close to her—she will nurture it and let it grow. She won't let anyone take it away from her. It is her rocket fuel and finally, she is going places. She can feel it down to her very core—this is her time. She will not only climb mountains—she will move them too.

Lang Leav
....

CHAPTER 5

Relationships, love, sex

To love a person is to see all their magic, and to remind them
of it when they have forgotten.

MARK GROVES

The relationship dance

Having my marriage to Cam somewhat played out in the media
as the 'perfect couple', I expect people must think it's been all
rainbows, love hearts and cupids singing us to sleep at night.

While there have been many moments like that, we've also
come incredibly close to leaving each other. I have loved, hated,
loved Cam more times than I can count. Each time we nearly
separated, we dug back in and grew. We learned a little more
about ourselves and each other and what love really looks and
feels like. What commitment means.

There is a dance that we do. Sometimes we dance together, sometimes apart, and sometimes—my least favourite—we dance until our toes are smashed by the other and we lie bleeding on the dance floor. Those dances can take a while to heal from and they usually require a bunch of kind-hearted women to carry you off the dance floor and bandage you up.

There is something really beautiful about being with someone from such a young age. We have been there for each other for so many life-changing experiences. So much history resides in our marriage. There are scars, sure, and there are patterns that still need tending to or else we find ourselves repeating behaviour that is just plain destructive.

Marriages fall apart for all sorts of reasons, and some really need to end. I feel fortunate to love someone so deeply and have that returned, and to know we were both willing to ride that rollercoaster together. I hate rollercoasters, by the way; I prefer the carousel, but that's relationships for you.

Me going through perimenopause has been another challenge for our marriage. We've faced harder experiences, as many long-term relationships often will, though this one did spin us both around for some time because of the way it affected our intimate and physical relationship. I'll explain how later in the book.

Potatoes

I know I'm feeling older than ever, my body shaping itself into an actual potato. And still I try to: Eat less! Exercise more! Urgh.

What if this potato shape is permanent? What if this is my final resting body shape?

Can I love this shape just as it is? How can we accept our bodies exactly as they are, in all their different and ever-changing forms?

How do I love my body when I hold the comparison to my 21-year-old self?

Feeling sexy is an inside job. I've recognised this as I have grown older. I'm not entirely comfortable with this realisation, I must admit, though I understand it from this perspective. When I asked myself when was the last time I felt sexy, I couldn't remember. It's been a very long time. Then I thought, 'Have I *ever* felt sexy?'

When you have been sexually assaulted, sexy becomes something that is dangerous. Feeling sexy under the male gaze is never going to be sustainable. Feeling sexy only when your partner compliments you and tells you how sexy you look is not sustainable. It's wonderful and lovely and can uplift your mood for a bit. But relying on the validation from men as to whether we are sexy or not is not only false but degrading.

If I don't believe that I'm sexy, the compliments start to roll like the proverbial water off a duck's back. I wish the equation was as simple as Cam x compliments = sexy. But for me, it's got to be more than that. The *more* I am still working on. Through the time of being in lockdown due to COVID-19 I felt more challenged than ever to find my sexy/sensual self, and I'm not sure if it was another phase of menopause, the stress of living in a world with a pandemic running riot or a combination of factors.

Freedom from the expectation of my own mind as to what I should look like is my end point. Self-love. Potatoes come in all shapes and sizes and are one of the most versatile vegetables. So maybe I'll start there.

Journal entry, September 2018

I'm worried, I've lost all desire for sex. I don't know what to do. I don't want to force myself to have sex with Cam. I feel trapped. Trapped in a body that feels . . . numb? What should I do? Is there a pill to get your libido back? Is there some hideous herbal drink that will make me want to rip my husband's clothes off and ravish him? Something that would feel consistent, not just a one-off? I feel embarrassment and shame coming up around not wanting sex. If I don't want it am I therefore no longer sexual? Am I not sexy? Is it my history of rape that has tainted my sexuality still to this day? Can I get past this sexual roadblock? I just feel nothing. It's not that I want any other man. I just don't want sex with any man. How do I get that desire back? I feel scared it's gone forever. I know Cam has said that without sex he won't stay. Panicked feelings arise in me as I think about him leaving, leaving because I can't be physically intimate with him. I feel the longer we don't have sex the more Cam goes numb, too, and gets frustrated at the same time. That he will turn off his desire for me in order to save himself. It's too easy to be lost in all the other symptoms that are louder—the aches and pains and hot flushes draw more attention than this empty feeling of loss. But in the quiet moments, that's when I feel afraid of what's gone. Fighting the darkness today, feeling the pull of sadness over this lack of intimacy. Feeling that I am to blame, that I am the one to somehow 'fix' myself. Am I broken? Did something break in me a long time ago and only now it's been driven to the surface? Right now, I don't know how to fix this. I guess I just need to start somewhere, start with a hug, hand holding, or a kiss. I need to get through my shame over not wanting to have sex to actually have sex. Breathe deep, breathe deep.

What makes conflict so painful is that we are desperate to be heard but too upset to listen, desperate to be understood but too upset to be understanding, desperate to be validated but too upset to be validating. What can help you get what you need is the willingness to stoke even a small ember of empathy for your partner's experience.

Alexandra Solomon
....

The penny dropped

One day, while conversing with a friend, she mentioned how her girlfriend was in perimenopause and how challenging it was for her. How their sex life had dwindled down to nothing and her girlfriend didn't even want to cuddle anymore. She said her girlfriend was too hot, prickly and angry a lot of the time. My friend was devastated, she felt pushed away and she was so concerned that their relationship had irrevocably changed for the worse.

Now I know what I'm about to write seems a tad unfair, but I heard that commentary as clear as day because it was a *woman* speaking about her girlfriend. Had a man been complaining about his wife and the lack of intimacy and sex, I would have risen with my feminist language in full tilt and said, 'How dare you, Sir. You have no idea what she's going through.' But when I heard this woman, I heard her pain and the loss that she was feeling. It clicked for me and I understood that our partners are struggling, too. For this I apologise to the men out there who are scratching their heads (and possibly their balls) at the sudden lack of sex and for not understanding that you, too, are in menopause with us.

I remember my husband looking at me in horror as I was mentioning to someone all my crazy symptoms, and that I don't know how long I'll feel this way, or how long my menopause will last—could be a few more years, or not.

He literally looked like someone had just thrown his golf bag off the Harbour Bridge. 'Years? Years? Are you kidding me? I can't handle years.'

Part (okay, most) of me (okay, all of me) wanted to scream, 'You have no clue.' This is not a choice I made. This would not be something I *would* choose, as a matter of fact. But it's here. We both have to deal with it. Well, in all honesty, he didn't have to do anything, he could walk away, he could ignore it, pretend it wasn't happening, or any number of other ways to deal with my menopause. In a perfect world I would have loved for Cam in that moment to be embracing, loving, tender, considerate about anything and everything I was feeling.

There's no rule book or emotional map for our partners in this game. When I wasn't wallowing in sweat and frustration I did feel for Cam and how our marriage was changing. I was not seeking any physical intimacy and I was so irritated . . . often with him.

The outcry

Will our male counterparts ever really understand menopause and what we are feeling? I don't know. Apparently women don't understand what getting kicked in the balls is like either. Men might only get kicked in the balls once in a lifetime, maybe never. Where do I start with women? Period cramps, endometriosis, labour pains, contractions, birth. Pap smears! Hello, forceps and tearing perineums. How do we describe menopause to our partners? I see Cam's eyes looking mighty confused when I talk about the grief and loss I've felt around my fertility.

'But you don't want any more kids,' he would say.

'I know. That's not the point,' I'd hurl back at him.

I know of women who have had a rough time needing to carry on with their regular work schedule while nursing multiple symptoms of perimenopause. How do you explain to your boss or co-workers that you can't focus, or need to walk out of meetings for fresh air as your temperature spikes. Menopause is one of the most underrated stressors for women who work. Yet we are expected to not only carry on, but not to complain, either.

How can I explain it in terms that a man might understand regarding the changes women go through both mentally and physically?

Say a man had worked hard all his life to own his own business, he loved his job, was successful, and then testosterone starts to slide. His hormones are taking a nosedive, he no longer can manage his business, he can only really work part time now, maybe doing some filing work and dusting around the office. His favourite suit no longer fits him due to weight gain for no apparent reason. He's lost some hair, his knees and elbows hurt and he becomes fairly invisible at the workplace. His penis is atrophying and sore, he feels tired all the time and people around him think he might be losing his mind. All because his body stopped producing the 'right stuff' to keep up with his job requirements.

Can you imagine if that happened to every man? Imagine the outcry! I wonder if there would be hundreds of tests, pills and potions all covered by healthcare for that?

Wouldn't it be wonderful if the men in our lives, our co-workers, our bosses, or employees, dads, brothers—all men—had an understanding about what menopause is actually about for us. To have empathy and support for us. That's a world I'd like to live in.

Sex

Would I have loved to feel like I wanted sex? Absolutely. The more I didn't have sex, the more guilty I felt. I'd lie in bed hoping that Cam was happy with a kiss and a lingering hand on his arm. I also know that he's not.

Physical intimacy is important. Emotional intimacy is important. I feel close to Cam when we've shared deep, meaningful, loving conversations—when I feel heard, when he's been curious about me, when we've discussed dreams and goals and we make plans together. Cam feels close by being physical, in all ways: lots of hugs and kisses and, of course, making love. So without that he feels lonely and separated from me; consequently, our emotional intimacy is affected, which alienates me. Round and round we go. It's often an easy fix. But it's getting past the 'who'll reach out first' hill that can make the separation drag on longer.

Because I felt so much anger as well during the worst of this time, the thought of sex was firmly tucked in the 'no way' box. I was too dang hot (and not in a good way) most of the time for touching, and sleep deprivation is the biggest killer of physical intimacy for me. I really wanted more than anything to feel different. Time and understanding, remedies and love have shifted this challenge in our marriage.

Talking about my symptoms and how I felt sexually with Cam was and has been helpful. I had to overcome the feeling of embarrassment that I had stopped wanting sex. When I was 100 per cent honest with Cam about everything, including my desire to get back my libido, we were able to tackle the issue together. I want to feel freedom with my body and mind in all ways, and a huge part of that is how I view myself as a sexual/sensual woman. Tackling this while in menopause, during a time when the last thing I wanted was to have sex, created a unique mix of challenges.

What I really wanted was to heal the sensual broken place I had been carrying inside for so long.

I highly recommend Dr Alexandra Solomon's book *Taking Sexy Back*. It's an eye-opening insight into many female sexual, sensual and intimacy issues. While reading it I discovered how long Cam and I had been in a shame-and-blame circle. He wanted sex because that was what he knew relationships were 'supposed to be built on', I felt pressured to live up to a certain amount of sex per week/month and, like a bad employee not fulfilling her tasks, I was failing. Cam blamed me for not wanting sex, I felt ashamed and embarrassed and from that point onward my libido was in hiding.

Taking Sexy Back explained all this and more, how as women we are sold a bill of goods about what sexy *is*, how it's often seen in external form, when in reality we need to feel our *internal* sexiness through ownership and love before we truly can enjoy sharing intimate space with someone else. Do yourself and your partner a favour and buy the book. It's a game changer.

Letter to my libido

Dear Libido,

Please come back, I miss you terribly. I promise to treat you better and pay more attention to you when you return. What is it that you need in order to return to me? Silk sheets? Erotic novels? Name it and I'll get it. Just please, come on home.

Love,
Me

Embracing this time in our lives I know is easier said than done. On my lowest of low days, I didn't want anyone to see me or speak to me. Even Cam. Actually, maybe even especially Cam. I struggled to find an answer to his question, 'What do you need?' What I wanted, what I *thought* I needed, was my fertility back, to stop burning up like I'd swallowed a volcano, to look in the mirror and *not* see a depressed, tired, fat, old woman. And I knew no one was going to hand that to me on a golden platter. Ever. Though asking for help with the kids, or my husband making dinner, made a small difference. Until I realised one day there was something I could ask for that would really help.

I asked my husband to not see me as someone who was broken and needed fixing. I didn't want to be looked upon with pity. I wanted him to remind me of my strength and my smarts, my beauty and my wisdom. I didn't want him to feel sorry for me in that I was starting perimenopause. I wanted him to help me see me as . . . well, still me—maybe a new and improved me—even when I couldn't. It wasn't until I verbalised this that I realised what I needed and he realised that there was a way he could help me. Up until then he felt a bit helpless and at a loss as to what to do.

We should not *ever* apologise to our partners for being in menopause. Our children never apologised for being in puberty. Both are natural processes.

We do need to understand, however, how our changes emotionally affect our families.

Ideally our partners shouldn't care if our brain has become a little foggy, or our skin is dry and itchy, and we should not be loved any less for our cranky mood swings or sweaty skin at odd times of the day and night. What I need to remember is that it can be all too easy to make Cam a target of my frustrations and mood swings. There is no clear message for him when I am in a dark, angry, sad place other than my communication becoming either non-existent or snappy. He begins to walk on the proverbial eggshells.

Patience with myself is key; taking a moment to breathe deep, especially if I feel I'm about to lash out at something completely irrelevant, such as, 'You bought Gala apples instead of Pink Ladies, you selfish bastard.'

The wrong apples are not a good cause for an emotional tongue-lashing.

Eight things that might help you and your partner keep the spark alive

1. Exercise. I know it sounds boring at times, and we hear this over and over, but a healthy body goes a long way to feeling sexy and sensual. Exercise can boost your mood like nothing else.
2. De-stress. Stress and sex are not great bedfellows. Find ways to unwind through meditation, long baths, candles—anything that helps you to unwind.
3. Head to your vitamin store and stock up on some zinc. It's an essential hormone balancer and assists the sex drive. You know the old wives' tale about eating oysters? Well, oysters are

full of zinc, so after the vitamin store, pop into your seafood market. Oysters also contain vitamin B_3, which assists with fatigue, which as we know can be a killer for your libido.

4. Depression. I understand this one. I don't believe you can feel depressed and sexually ready at the same time. Seek help for your depression the best way possible and your sex life will also benefit.

5. Need I mention how important the 'S' word is? Yep, you guessed it: SLEEP. My goodness, sleep is everything when it comes to libido and sexual desire. So find ways to get your zzzzzz's.

6. Find out what turns you on. You may have been in a relationship where your focus was solely on your partner's needs. What makes you put the brakes on lovemaking? And what makes your accelerate? Open discussion with your partner about how, when and where you want to make love can turn up the heat (in a good way this time).

7. Cut out what lowers your libido. Things like smoking, drug use and excessive alcohol have all been shown to lower sex drive.

8. Try something new together. Take risks, plan adventures, learn a new language or how to cook Thai food together. Learning something together can open up some great conversation and intimacy that may just lead you to the bedroom.

For you, the bedfellow

One of the goals of this book is to assist partners of menopausal women. By:

1. helping them to understand what we are feeling
2. helping them with how to support us
3. letting them know they might need support too

Can I say—I think partners really need help. I know my husband does. It's not just me going through menopause, it's everyone who lives with me. We can be a wonderful tricky lot, us women—I know I am. I have trouble with being as clear about what I need from Cam. When my hormones are also in overdrive, not only am I up shit creek without a paddle, I'm too tired and irritated to row back to my husband and call out for help, which causes a rift between us.

Communication is key. It's also what can get so lost between couples. Cam and I have done hours of therapy and tending to our marriage, and yet still there can be a chasm between us. Especially when I can't figure out all these new emotions and bodily sensations. I also recognise that in talking with Cam about menopause, I have felt less attractive to him. I've wanted to hide it (impossible). I've wanted to run from the feelings (also impossible) because of my own beliefs around menopause being a negative occurrence. Mainly because that's what we women have been fed. For years and years, that's all I've heard. I so want to change that, for myself, for my daughters and for all women . . . and actually men, too.

It was after I had another dark couple of months during perimenopause that Cam suggested we see a counsellor together.

I was just so angry, sad and in a spin thinking my marriage was over, I thought I no longer loved my husband and started figuring out ways to divorce, keep the children, have a home, work. I told no one of the depths of thoughts and feelings as they seemed so unreal for me. I loved my husband, didn't I?

I came from a divorced family and truly didn't want to repeat that pattern. Yet I would lie awake at night having heart palpitations about needing to get away from the life we currently lived. It was like I'd opened some surreal Pandora's box and every little hurt, real or imagined, came pouring out. I was suddenly mad for things that happened years and years ago. Things we had talked through and worked through with heartfelt apologies. It was like the wounds were still fresh.

Cam, of course, was totally confused. Our love life was absolutely non-existent. I could barely manage a kiss. I was not sleeping in the same bed. I felt relief when he was not home. Communication had come to a stop; any time we attempted to talk, I was infuriated by what I felt was his total lack of understanding and care. I was mad at him for everything.

Cam was the one to suggest a counsellor. He was surprised when I so readily said, 'Yes'. I think he was expecting me to say, 'We're fine, we can work it out'. I knew I needed a third party. I knew I couldn't say everything that was rattling around in my brain, as I knew it would be the end of our marriage.

I also knew all these thoughts weren't exactly logical.

Within three sessions I started feeling so much better. Having the safety of a good therapist in the room with you helps an enormous amount. My brain stopped spinning and dragging up 'hurt files' from twenty years ago. I could see my husband again; I could hear him again.

Hormonal shifts can be mind-boggling in their intensity and their highs and lows. I'm so grateful that there was that little part of me that hung in there and that I can feel how much I am still in love with the man I married.

A big clue for me about the thoughts I was having around my husband, feeling like the marriage was over, that I no longer loved him, was that those perceptions came about when I was at the height of my mood swings, when my symptoms were on fire. So I could grasp that there was a connection between my hormones and my exaggerated thinking around Cam. That was a relief.

I mentioned to an older gentleman that I was writing a book about menopause and joked that it will be a book he will never have an interest in. His response surprised me. He said, 'I wish I had a book like you're writing when my wife was going through menopause. We couldn't make it work through that time and I was lost as to how to help her. We've been divorced fifteen years now.'

Not the first or last time that I've heard divorce enter the picture while the wife is dealing with menopause.

A good friend had a hell of a time with perimenopause; her husband really struggled at the time, not knowing how to support his wife. When I mentioned I was writing a book that I hoped would support the partners of women as well as the women he was so thrilled that there was something he could read that might make a difference to their relationship.

It's sometimes so hard to step back a little and see that what we are going through affects others, especially when we feel so incredibly consumed by our own feelings. I found it helpful for me when I was in an upswing, a good head space and balanced, to have those talks with Cam. To let him know that what I'm feeling may seem nuts, crazy, hysterical, confusing.

Not knowing yourself as you swing like a pendulum from one emotion to the next is incredibly disconcerting. As it can be for our loved ones.

What does my partner need?

Can I even get to that question? Can I make enough space to ask it and then see if there is enough room to accommodate his needs?

Prepare for menopause together, so you can tackle any issue as a united front.

Ladies, here is the section where I recommend you pass the book over to your significant other. Pass it with love and gentleness. It's not very long—don't worry. I hope this section makes a difference to you both and that some kind of conversation and understanding comes forth.

My wife is going through menopause. Everyone speaks of the women. What about the men these women are married to? It's so hard for husbands trying to deal with a menopausal woman. It's been six years that we've been dealing with it. I'm ready to leave her. I can't deal with the non-stop arguing, smart mouth, and blaming me for everything. I'm drained and feel like I'm going to have a nervous breakdown.

YouTube quote
....

Dear Partners of Menopausal Women,

Hello and welcome aboard what could possibly feel like The Crazy Train. The ride could be rough, it will be bloody hot and sometimes freezing cold. Buckle in. We are on a journey and, yes, you're coming with us. There may be roadblocks, separate beds, tears (almost a guarantee). But there is an end to all this.

If you could be so kind as to hang in there with us, you may really love the final destination. A wonderful, feisty, creative, honest woman.

Here's something to keep in mind as often as you can recall it. Women can seem complicated, but at the end of the day we just want to be loved and heard. I know you need the same thing from us, too. I know you need to talk about the challenges of living with us as well. That the wife or partner you married might seem different now. I get it. Depending on where your partner is at, she may not be the best person to talk with about all those items. Maybe she is, in her quieter, cooler moments, then talking to her without blaming would be a positive thing.

Remember there are many ways to feel close to your partner: rather than sex being a same-old, one-course meal, offer a banquet! If your partner does not feel like sex, offer her to just lay in your arms, or ask if she would like a foot rub. Get creative about how you can still have intimacy, though with one main point: let her know that this foot massage, or cuddle on the couch, does not mean you then are *owed* sex.

Let the intimacy build, let her simply feel you, feel loved by you, without the pressure of sex.

I've created a blueprint for intimacy for you partners out there based on what I need to hear from my husband. Obviously use your own words, and if you already know how to speak to your partner with healing, kind words, amazing! Maybe you could share your knowledge with a friend whose relationship might be strained from the changes their wife is going through.

My husband can be at a loss at knowing what to say when I am at a low point about my body or my life in general. He is a Mr Fixit Dude, and when I'm emotional he slightly panics as to what are the best words to say. He just wants to know the 'right' words that will bring his wife closer to him once more. Can you relate to that?

Repartee

Okay, here's an example of one conversation with my husband. This is how *not* to respond.

ME: I wish I could wear shorts, but I can't anymore. My legs look like they kind of melted, they just seemed to have gone to mush overnight. My legs are ugly.

HUSBAND: But you are doing exercise, right? They shouldn't look like that?

ME: I don't get it. I don't understand a lot of my body right now. I've been doing exercise, but they just seem to be getting more flabby.

HUSBAND: (Cue silence for two long minutes.) So, what do you want for dinner?

You know what happened after that? I was hurt, sad and felt like the ugliest human on earth.

You know how my husband felt? Utterly confused and panicked because he didn't know the right words to say and knew he'd put his foot in his mouth again but felt nothing he could say would make any difference anyway.

Now I *know* we can't look for outside validation. I *know* that our beauty comes from how we feel about ourselves, I *know* that we don't need a man/woman to tell us we are beautiful. I also *know* that I do want my husband to find me attractive and offer some support while I'm feeling so incredibly crappy.

So, let's try this again, shall we? How about this for a supportive dialogue.

ME: I wish I could wear shorts, but I can't anymore. My legs look like they kind of melted, they just seemed to have gone to mush overnight. My legs are ugly.

HUSBAND: Honey, you can wear anything and I still love you. I love your legs, always have, always will.

ME: I don't get it. I don't understand a lot of my body right now. I've been doing exercise, but they just seem to be getting more flabby.

HUSBAND: It must be really challenging for you and what you are feeling. If there is anything I can do to help you, let me know. We will get through this together. Just know that I love you and I always see you as beautiful.

Annnnnnnd end scene.

Does that seem doable? It's pretty simple. But wow, does it make a world of difference when we feel like you are present with us in this crazy experience.

Okay, look. How to compliment a menopausal woman may actually be harder than swimming the English Channel one-armed and blindfolded. One day the compliment you are giving seemed fine and the next day she may look at you with a total death stare.

For example, another conversation with my husband:

CAM: You're getting your body back.

ME: What, so I'd lost it before?

CAM: Well, you were the one who said you were fat and bloated, I'm just saying you're getting your body back. It's great.

ME: (Internally thinks: My body *back*? What if I didn't lose weight? Why is it great I'm looking like I did before?

Why can't it be okay that I am the shape I am now? The pressure is always to keep the youthful figure. Instead, I swallow and say . . .) Thanks.

I know Cam is attempting a compliment here. I'll take it on its intent, him saying something nice. But what would have been some alternative words to 'you're getting your body back' that might have been a bit more digestible?

How about:

- You look so strong and beautiful, how do you feel? I get excited every time I see you.
- Your mind is just as sexy as your beauty. I love every inch of you.
- You look beautiful even when you don't try. You have the sweetest heart.
- I love looking at you.
- You are always beautiful to me. I want you to see how beautiful you are, too.

Love language

As my body changed I had so much difficulty finding acceptance and beauty in what I saw reflected back at me in my mirror. I had convinced myself that my husband also saw me as unattractive. He promised me he in fact did not see the ugly that I saw. He tells me he finds me more beautiful now. Some days I still feel unconvinced. Those days I feel sad that I cannot believe what he's telling me. I say this to you (dear partner, of menopausal woman) as you may be experiencing the same thing with your significant other, how she is seeing herself as ugly, unlovable, and far from sexy. All of those feelings make for a very challenging experience related to any sensual relationship with you.

She is possibly feeling the stress and anxiety that may come with shifting hormones, and that includes exhaustion and brain fog, which can cause stress in itself when she is at work or home and being the person that 'always remembers and organises everything'. Add to that the anxiety around her evolving body shape and worry about her lack of interest in sex and it's an entire package of stress. She needs understanding and your love more than anything.

This is where you may need to dig deep into your love language. For example, what can you compliment your partner on?

- Do the complimenting in public.
- Tell people how beautiful you find her—now more than ever.
- Tell people and her how age suits her, that she is wise and an amazing wife/mother/sister/daughter.
- Tell her, because her self-esteem may have been rocked to such a degree she can't see herself clearly.

Having someone on her side pointing out the beauty of her, inside and out, is a gift that will stay with her forever. It might take a while to crack through the wall of self-defeat and the nasty critic in her head, but please give it your best and see what magic comes from it.

Passing along information I've found on the internet to Cam has been helpful. So he can read up on what's going on not just for me, but for millions of other women. It was important for Cam to understand it was not just me feeling all these emotions and symptoms but a whole bevy of women worldwide going through almost the exact same experience. Now we can find small moments together that are still sweet, like walking the dogs, or holding hands while watching a movie. I can explain that sometimes sleeping separately is to *save* the marriage, not because I *hate* the marriage. (That was a helpful sentence; I had to repeat that a fair few times before Cam understood.) It's not been easy with Cam, I am the first to admit it. We did vow to love each other in sickness and in health. Staying patient with myself and with him is so important right now.

And now a word or two from my sponsor . . . actually, my husband.

Cam

Regarding menopause, I knew nothing. My mother never really broached the subject with me; I was well out of the family home by the time she reached menopause. I recall my sister's complaints that Mum was going through a tough time of change and that her patience was thin, however I am still not clear today whether she was referring to Mum's patience with her, or her patience for my mum. My sister never spoke of it either. So given that the most influential women in my life never spoke of it, I never thought to ask beyond what I'd picked up from a magazine in the dentist's office.

I've found the best way to assist Ali is to . . . listen to her. Your partner may not want to talk, but remain open and ready to listen when she does. I try not to take things personally. For me, that's a tough one. Her menopause is not about me, and it is always in my best interests to keep it with her, instead of making it about what I am not getting.

Ali is evolving into an even more beautiful woman and this is being driven from the inside. Her intuitive side has evolved to new levels of understanding. In other words, she knows and calls me on my bullshit from a much greater distance. And her willingness to put up with bullshit from me or others has dwindled as much as those damn hot flushes have continued to bubble through her glowing skin.

I have seen her intention to be fit and healthy take action in ways I have never seen before; I have also seen her deal with her body changing in ways that are counterintuitive to what she is intending. I totally understand her frustration when she comes downstairs from the bedroom completely flustered that a pair of jeans she just bought no longer fit.

To me she has become as beautiful and shapely, as she is strong and vulnerable.

So how can you support your woman through menopause?

It can be a challenging time for partners as well, as so much might be changing. Not only for your partner emotionally and physically, but within your relationship, As her partner, believe me, you can help. Research shows that taking the time to read up on and understand menopause for yourself is a great form of support. When she's feeling unusually sensitive about a subject you will know it's just her hormones. Your knowledge about menopause can make a big difference for the both of you. The more you know, the more ways you can support her. Having a partner who understands that menopause and all its symptoms might be wreaking havoc on your wife, and not taking it personally, is the best medicine a gal can have.

Here are some tips that might help you both.

Talk about it

Letting your partner know that you are there to listen and talk about what she is experiencing is a great way to support her, whatever her mood. That kind of support can shift and improve her wellbeing and assist her to cope with the symptoms.

Your partner's menopausal symptoms affect you, too. Make sure she knows that you're in this together and you are doing your best to understand how she feels.

Remember, menopause doesn't last forever. I promise, eventually the symptoms will subside. If you do have concerns for your partner, maybe offer a gentle suggestion that she see a doctor, therapist, whomever could help her most. You are on the outside looking in, and you may just be the best person to notice how hard a time your partner is having. Suggesting a doctor's visit shows how much you care. Going with her to the appointment would be a beautiful show of solidarity.

Understand that your partner may not want sex

Oh boy, this is a tough one. I think, of all the challenges in a relationship that menopause may bring, the lack of sex can drive a wedge bigger than anything.

I can't say this enough: when your partner says, 'I don't want sex', it doesn't mean she doesn't want you.

One of the symptoms of menopause can be a change in sex drive. Trust me, the hormones might be spiking or dropping like a rollercoaster, so sex is sometimes the last thing on our minds. It can be just as devastating to us as it is to you. Don't take it personally, it's not about you.

Midlife stresses brought on by career changes, the loss of a loved one, empty nest syndrome or caring for elderly parents can also contribute to a declining libido.

Throw in how she feels about her changing body, and the undeniable pressure woman are under to 'look good', well, your partner may just be in survival mode, and be in no mood to connect physically.

You might need to take it back to good old G-rated romance: spending quality time together, finding new ways to connect. Hold hands while walking on the beach, have dinner by candle-light. All that good stuff we did when we were younger, while romancing our loves. Think of this time as a way to bring you even closer—try some new things: hobbies, weekends away. Show her you are doing the best you can to understand her and all her symptoms.

As you and your partner age, there are shifts occurring for both of you. Your partner's changes may look a little different to yours. The production of male hormones generally declines very gradually, usually less than one per cent a year after the age of 30 or so. Having hormonal shifts in common may just be the connection that you've been looking for! Snap.

Men in the 40–50 age range do note that they sometimes have:

- reduced physical strength
- a degree of muscle loss
- mood swings and irritability
- loss of libido
- erectile dysfunction
- changes in sleep patterns
- reduced energy
- depressed mood
- lack of motivation.

Mental health for both of you at this time is so important. If you are experiencing any of these symptoms, make sure there is not an underlying health issue. It may be as simple as testosterone decline. Men are often in denial about their symptoms, they have an 'it will get better' or 'she'll be right' attitude. Making a date at the doctor for the both of you might just be a lifesaver.

When we love another, we face our shit. We face our limitations. We see where we lack skills. We see how bad our communication can be. We feel our reactivity and our sense of unworthiness. When we turn towards love, towards a human who sees our light and wants to love us deeply, we experience what it means to face a feeling we have not felt worthy of for some time . . . if not our whole lives. To love is easy. To be loved requires the belief we're worthy of it . . . and the only way to feel worthy is to allow yourself to be.

Mark Groves

....

Letter to my husband

Dear Husband of 28 Years,

I'm still me. I might look, sound, react differently than I ever have. I may jump at the smallest of things and cry literally over spilt milk, I may worry about the state of the earth till I'm bedridden, or feel that my life has come to an abrupt end. I may even say I have nothing to live for or that no one understands me. I know these things are hard to hear. I know you must be thinking: What about me? I'm still here, I'm your friend. Why can't she get over this? Don't I wish I could.

Those kinder, gentler days when I would bend over backwards for you and the kids, put everything aside to make sure everyone was happy; those days of spending nearly every second thinking what more could I do to make you happy, make sure your career, your joy, your life was top notch; those days when I said, 'I'll do it, I'm fine, I'll take care of it'—those days are behind me and you now. And they need to be.

I know I've trained you well to lean on me for so many things, I know I've put you first above so many of my own needs, and I know this may be a confusing time for you as I upend the raft and tip us both into the river. But I have to, I need to and I want to. I'm doing my best to not blame you for everything, large and small. To walk away and breathe when I want to scream till my eyes bulge from my head. I know sometimes you see me attempting to keep all these feelings at a decent level. I'm not sorry for going through menopause. I'm not sorry for changing and growing. I'm not sorry for evening out the scales of importance. I'm just sorry it's taken me this long.

Now I can't hold back these feelings anymore and, as they rush in, it takes both of our breaths away. I am sorry for when I don't see how hard you are trying to be kind and understanding, or when you reach for a hug and I stiffen in your arms. I know you need love like I do; I can barely keep up with all the feelings. I know you are simply being swept up in my tailwind. But this is me for right now, honey, in sickness and in health, hot and cold. I love you. Thank you for loving me.

Love,
Me

Relationship with yourself

Journal entry, February 2019

It's been days of feeling the same: itchy skin, irritable, sad, teary, angry, frustrated, sleepless and hot.

I want to be alone, yet I feel lonely. I want total silence and yet I want people to call me. I want to not be touched and yet I want physical connection. My mum rubbed my aching back the other day and I nearly wept from the feel of her hand.

I want nothing to do, yet I want a purpose. I want freedom from my thoughts—rattling, repetitive thoughts—yet I want to figure out who and what I want for my future. I want no responsibility, yet I look at young mums with their toddlers and I'm desperate to have that time back again. I want to scream, but I don't want to talk.

I want to stop pushing, pushing to get up, keep moving, see the bright side, reach out to others, yet I know I must—this is my passage through. I want to feel wise, yet I feel old.

What does living life to the fullest even mean? And following my dreams?

My whole life was centred around, geared for, counting the days till I had children. That was my dream.

It came true three times and it was better and harder than I ever could have imagined. So now what?

Menopause as a launch pad

Menopause has made me realise that it's not my body that's the problem, it's the way I think about my body. I've been brainwashed from a young age that skinny is better, cellulite is bad, size small is sexy. That there is shame in our bodies if they step outside of the perfect shape, that I should feel embarrassed to wear a bikini at my age—only one-pieces for the over-fifties! It's been hard to love my body and the changes that it's going through when the message from society is that I shouldn't.

I've officially kissed goodbye to all the clothes I've clung to that don't fit anymore. Formerly tucked away, wrapped in hope that one day I might actually wear them again. I felt sad about letting them go—it's letting go of a dream, really—but they tended to keep me wanting, wanting to look different than I do. Judging of the weight I'd gained. Every now and again when I felt I'd lost a little weight I would attempt to slide a pair of pants on, only to be devastated that the zip *still* did not close. Yeah, it was time to not only let the clothes go but also the pressure to fit in them as well.

Journal entry, April 2019

I feel woefully unprepared for this middle-aged life where my children are nearly fully grown and so independent. The adjustments are hard.

More so because I'm truly left with all this time . . . time for what, I ask? Myself? Well, isn't that a foreign concept!

*My body is really talking right now. And its voice is
LOUD, louder than it's ever been. I'm listening—I have to,
I need to, because it's racked up a lot to say.*

The emotions surrounding my cycle coming to an end and therefore no longer being able to become pregnant have been the hardest to grapple with. What I don't have, what is missing now, has dredged up so many memories of my children as babies, everything from their miraculous births to their first steps, to long nights breastfeeding. I loved it all. I miss it all. Now, I have this feeling that something was taken from me without my permission.

There is this imagery I've read about with women and the phases of their lifetime. Do you know 'Maiden, Mother and Crone'? I don't want to be the 'Crone'. I know the 'Crone' is a representation of a women with wisdom, but can they stop drawing her as a wizened old lady in a cape and hood with a walking stick? I did not sign up for that. I did not audition—nope, not me.

To add to this, herein lies a tricky part of menopause for some of us. If you have had children, often, as you are hitting menopause, your child is into their teens or older. I have a 24, 20 and fourteen- soon to be fifteen-year-old. So those baby years are long gone for all three. Their independence is cemented. So, the empty nest is coinciding with an empty uterus. It may seem illogical, I don't actually *want* more children, but I don't want my ability to have children to be gone either. Men can impregnate a woman till they are at least 60 and even beyond. I may just plan a march with my placard and say, 'Equal Fertility Rights for Women'!

For me, my career has been being a mother; I chose to stay at home and raise my three, often on my own as Cam has travelled extensively for work. So now I feel . . . redundant. I'm not ready to surrender my name tag, give up my preferred parking space and Christmas bonus. Mothering does feel more part-time/casual work these days. And I know in my heart of hearts that this, this piece right here, this empty space left by the ghost of my life with small children, is where the beginning of *my* independence starts.

I'm floundering a little, sure. 'What am I going to *do* with the rest of my life?' is a recurring question. But there is excitement in this newfound sense of time for *me*.

What I also know is that I need time to grieve. I want to give myself the time, as long as I need, to feel sad about my fertility. It's the end of a beautiful chapter. But not the end of the book. I want to celebrate that time, too. Acknowledge all that it took to raise children, juggle a million different things and all the while stay loving and present for my babies. Congratulate the body that birthed them, fed them, and held their hands. Because only then I can feel the possibilities of my next chapter. I can love the space that is solely mine to step into. CEO of me.

Do you have that feeling?

Unshackling

A point of contention in my marriage to Cam has been that I've believed he's done everything he's wanted to do while I've remained at home taking care of everything related to our home life. I truly convinced myself that I couldn't go off on my own and do things I longed to do. I had, over the course of our marriage, given up—little piece by little piece—on my own needs and dreams. I was, instead, a wife and a mother first and foremost—a somewhat vanilla version of myself that at times felt hard done by, because of what I had to sacrifice.

But when I think about it, Cam was constantly offering to take care of the kids, for me to go away if I wanted to, to spend time doing the things I once loved, but did I? Not for a very long time. I felt I couldn't, I felt so guilty for even wanting to have a break. I absolutely loved what I had; being a mum and a wife was my ultimate dream, so therefore I should be there for my family 24/7, right?

I'm incredibly proud of my children and the longevity of my marriage. I've worked hard at doing the best that I could for my family. But there is an important part of the family dynamic that was not tended to for a long time: Me. What did I want?

So, what of this new feeling? This freedom? I am surprised and slightly horrified that I want to put myself at equal first. Menopause and middle age seems to have heralded this new sense of myself. I had been indoctrinated through multiple cultural examples that I, as a woman and a mother, should be low on my own list of importance, that I should show the kindness of my soul by sacrificing myself to others. I wear a badge of honour by being exhausted from taking care of others.

Now as I shift into my 'me zone', how do I begin to be okay with finding myself first in line? It's exhilarating and most definitely undeveloped. Is this okay? Is it alright that I leave the room and close the bedroom door for an hour to read my book and drink tea in peace? That I step back from the constant expectation that Mum will cook, clean, shop, take care of the house? Cam and I have our agreed-upon roles: Cam the breadwinner, Ali the homemaker. And now I want to tear those roles to shit. In fact, I've been feeling more than a little suffocated by that role. In the same way that Cam feels bound to always be the breadwinner. I crave to have not just a day, a week, but a length of time that feels right for me where all I think about is *me*. Is that evil? Is that ugly and narcissistic? The good girl people pleaser is completely horrified, but she's no longer the loudest voice in my head. The loudest voice is seductive and she calls on me to say, *Yes*—be you, go for it, unshackle the role you've been in.

I'm like a runaway train. The good girl, I hope, will never rule the roost again.

I do my best to explain this new feeling coursing through me to Cam. He seems worried at what that might mean for him, for us. Do I want to leave and have an *Eat Pray Love* experience? No. Maybe. Not sure. Yes. Absolutely not. I fantasise about what it would be like to not think about making sure kids get to school, that lunches are ready, shopping is done, dinner hot and ready on the table; what would it be like to be done with all that, so I am free and clear to wander through my day asking myself, 'So what do you want to do?' It's new territory, so I have no road map for it. I do know I need to communicate with Cam about all of this. I also know I need this; I want this.

Friendships with women

Friendships can be lifesavers. If you have a group of friends, I'm sure you already know that.

Having a supportive circle of women who are experiencing similar feelings or at least willing to listen to you is healing and helpful. Any self-help book or therapist will most likely say that a woman's social support network during menopause greatly influences her quality of life. We are most open with those who are willing to listen empathetically and share some truths of their own.

Beware of the friends you feel more depressed around. Ones that dismiss how you feel and want you to just 'get over it'.

Use menopause to create a closeness with other women, swap handy hints, talk about the symptoms and challenges, share details of alternative medicines or any doctors that have assisted you. Swap recipes and the name of the yoga studio you attend. And, of course, share your funny, light-hearted and positive stories.

Organise walks together, or start a new hobby, have a revolving dinner party once a month, create a book club. Keep searching for ways to connect with like-minded women.

Not everyone is fortunate enough to have a group of friends; you may have lost touch with them, or like me you might have moved countries and need to start making friends all over again. It can be incredibly challenging, but also rewarding. I found that the effort had to come from me. Everyone around me already had a friendship group, so it was up to me to get the ball rolling . . . and keep it rolling until the invites started coming my way.

Adult education classes are always a good way to meet people of a similar age. My favourite way to meet like-minded people is to volunteer for something I am passionate about. Seek out your women friends; they are looking for you, too.

There is nothing better than a friend, unless it is a friend with chocolate.

Linda Grayson
....

For the kids

While we are at it, you may have some other people in your sphere at home with you. I have three children, and they are also going through menopause with me, whether they like it or not. How much does my twenty-year-old son want to talk about Mum's menopause?

I'd say about as much as he wants to clean his room and feed the dogs.

It's surprising how many children remember their mum going through 'something' at around the 48 to 50-year mark. Again, if I am feeling confused and frustrated about the changes I'm experiencing, for sure my kids do not know why the hell I freak out about them not replacing the toilet paper, or why I may look at them and burst into tears and suddenly talk about when they were little and how they used to love being with me.

The mum that was super happy to be cooking and cleaning, taxi-driving kids around, and not raising her voice, may have disappeared. The mum who can't 'cook one more meal this week or I'll lose my shit' may have moved in.

How do we talk to our kids about menopause?

For me, always honestly and without a lecture that goes any longer than five minutes. You know that feeling when you've lost the attention of your kids: the squirming, the eye rolling, the reaching for the phone. Short and honest, I say.

With the most important part of the 'talk' being these words: 'This is not about you.'

You may need to repeat those words over and over.

Once they know that I am not cranky at them for being alive, that I am personally going through something challenging, that I love them all the same, and I will handle everything I feel, they are free to move about the cabin. Safety has been established again.

Letter to my kids

Dear Children,

Your mum is doing the best she can. These physical and emotional changes she is going through are not easy. You may see her crying more (not about you); you may hear her yelling more (not about you); you may see her really sad (not about you). She may seem extra picky and what was okay last week when you had three dirty glasses in your room may seem now like you murdered Bambi (not about you, though it would really help if you did in fact put your bloody cups in the dishwasher).

So how can you help? What action can you take if you want to support your mum at this time? Well, it's patience. Patience like when she waited for three hours to watch you play sport, or waited in the dentist's office. Patience while you threw up all over her from that virus and she rubbed your back. Remember all the kind things and know it's the same lady under all that sweat.

Love,

Me

Things you can say:

- Need a hand with the dishes, Mum?
- Need some help with dinner?
- Do you want me to get you more ice/an ice pack?
- You look great, Mum!

And the Number 1 bestseller . . .

- I love you.

Kids, it's a passing phase. Ask questions if you need more info. Mum is not sick or dying. Mum is making some changes and the growth period is just a little, well . . . prickly.

Mothers and daughters

I have two daughters. My eldest is more like me—extremely sensitive and somewhat anxious. She's also a people pleaser like me; I watch her rebuff compliments and judge her own wisdom, and it drives me absolutely nuts because she is my reflection, she is the sum of society's pressure and her mother's demonstration.

My youngest, however, didn't get the memo. She is confident; she will tell you how great she is; she will own her prowess at dancing, writing, singing. And you know what? I watch it land on people and I watch people struggle with it—this young lady of fourteen having all that confidence, how dare she!

She's been called arrogant, cocky, and told she 'needs to be taken down a peg'. I used to worry for her emotional safety when I heard her declare how bloody fabulous she is.

I would think, 'You can't say that.' Why? Because people won't like you.

Wrong. Hell no. You can say whatever you like about the fabulousness of yourself. If other people have a problem, that's on them.

Here in Australia, where the tall poppy syndrome still exists, can women dare to be seen as leaders, as confident, or will they be seen as aggressive and too masculine?

Understanding this has created wonderful conversations with both of my daughters. With my eldest I apologised for what I taught her, and what social media has put in her brain. I'm so grateful to be able to speak and have her comprehend these conversations, she's smart and beautiful and sensitive. I have total faith that she will come to understand herself quicker than her mother has done.

And I spoke to my youngest and told her that under no circumstances is she to change. That her confidence is her superpower. She's at that age where other girls' opinions are just beginning to make an impact on her. The beginning of wanting to fit in, of dumbing down, adjusting, submitting, acquiescing.

Sharing with my youngest that when she is 100 per cent authentic it gives an example to her friends to do the same, I see her eyes widen; that hits her. Truly, though, she is as much my example as I am to her. I know how important her self-confidence is. And I know I'm growing into mine.

My mother is one of the sweetest ladies I know. We talk about anything and everything now—not so much when I was growing up. I'm sure I was somewhat of the regular teenage girl who didn't think to ask their mum about growing old or our place in the world. Now, we've had so many important conversations. Menopause being one of them. Encouraging the younger generation to be everything they want to be is a gift we give them and ourselves.

Another letter to my children

My Beautiful Kids,

Thank you for riding this wave with me, for not teasing me or laughing when I would run from the room in a boiling hot sweat. For offering me ice packs for the back of my neck. For telling (lying to) me about how I have not gained weight. For encouraging me to 'go out, have fun'. For being so patient when I yet again talked about menopause. If you had a dollar every time I mentioned *that* word, you'd be set for life. You are the best.

Love,
Your Red-hot Mum xo

CHAPTER 6

Changing, adapting, realigning

It's through times of great change that I have found the
beautiful constants in my life. I will always be grateful.

SOULFULPENGUIN

Journal entry, April 2019

*Fat, feel fat, fat as fuck, I eat I get fat, I don't eat I get fat,
I exercise I get fat. Fat as fuck. Meant to love all this fat,
but I don't; meant to love this shape I'm in, but I don't; meant
to embrace myself and all that I am, but I don't. I'm fat, tired
of seeing it, feeling it, knowing it, hating it. Fat. Too much
pressure to not be fat, too many messages to not be fat. Tired of
the messages, tired of the beliefs, tired of my beliefs about my
own body. Can I love the fat I'm in? Not today, Motherfucker.
Maybe tomorrow, next week? Not today. Today I want to whine
and curse and complain and hide my fat. I think it's trying to*

get my attention. This fucking fat of mine. If I listen to my
fat, what does it say? I'm here to stay? I see my mother's body
looking back at me. I love my mother but I'm at war with my
body that looks more and more like hers every day. How can I
judge my own and not hers?

Menopause belly

I'm standing in line at my local post office. I approach the counter to ask for some stamps and to post a package, and the well-meaning post office clerk's eyes travel downwards to my belly and up again, and she asks me in an excited voice, 'How far along are you?'

I've had to deal with this before. Inwardly, I groan.

'I'm not pregnant,' I say.

The clerk looks to the customer in the next line. 'But you must be,' she says as she waves vaguely in the direction of my stomach.

'Nope, just fat.'

As bad as I felt, I think the post office clerk felt worse. Maybe I shouldn't have used the term 'just fat', maybe I could have explained that my hormones had plummeted, I was not sleeping, and I was stressed, so my middle had grown exponentially. Instead, I told her, 'It's okay, don't feel bad,' and took my change and my pregnant-looking belly with me.

I would love to tell you that I love my body all the time, but as yet I can't. Some days I feel the small flames of love or at least acceptance for the changes, though on average I don't dwell too long looking in the mirror or lavish praise upon my naked being. There is an expectation, especially for women, that the goal is to look in the mirror and feel unconditional love, body positivity. I would sing Hallelujah from the rooftops if all women, and why not men as well, could feel that kind of love. Sometimes, though, that feels unrealistic and only adds to more pressure around how we should feel. And I'm so sick and tired of anyone telling me how I should feel about my physical body, including myself.

What I'm in the process of learning is gratitude for my body. 'Look like a celebrity' diets and exercise routines drive me bonkers. My body does not look anything like it did when I was fourteen or at 38, it's been continually changing since I was born, and who said we should look like our eighteen-year-old self? Probably me, now, come to think of it . . . Sigh.

Have I embraced my new shape? That's a work in progress. Bottom line is, I've never been satisfied with my shape, so judging my body parts is not new. Dear belly, it's you I'm having trouble loving. It's you that seems to grow no matter what I do or eat, or not eat.

I did however have this epiphany in yoga a while ago. I lay there at the end on my mat with my hands on my belly, the belly that has weathered so much, and I felt sorry for all the hate I've thrown its way, all the pinching of fat that I do while I exclaim, 'So disgusting'. I thought about how much my belly does for me each and every day. I began to have a feeling of love. Love for the belly, the overhang. Love.

Maybe give the same thoughts to your belly a whirl. Maybe you love your belly already, but if you don't, just quietly lie there with your hands on your tummy like you would place your hands on a baby and feel whatever you feel. Hopefully you will experience positive feelings. If not, stop. No need to keep punishing yourself if you are not in the right headspace or heart space. I get that. Maybe the yoga brought it on for me, maybe I wouldn't have had the same experience had I simply lay down in my house with my dogs licking at my face and the dirty dishes in the sink. Whatever the scenario, feeling love towards my belly was and continues to be a new-found feeling.

Something I will revisit often as I waver back and forth between judgement and kindness.

Letter to my muffin top

Dear Muffin Top,

Look, I get why you are hanging around. I stretched the crap out of you with the pregnancies and then I overate and pretty much stopped using my stomach muscles for eleven years. Just so you know, you are now free to leave. It's not you, it's me. I'm ready to fit into my pants again, you see, and I really want to be stopped being asked if I'm pregnant. I'm sorry if I couldn't love you the way I should. I just want to have a waist again. Part of you will most likely always be with me, I can deal with that. I'd really love to start seeing other body parts. Like my vagina.

Love,

Me

To love yourself and everyone and everything in your life, is to give yourself heaven right now and ensure your place there for eternity.

Alan Cohen
....

Brain fog

My memory's not as sharp as it used to be. Also, my memory's not as sharp as it used to be.

I heard the other day that we humans are programmed to be fearful of change. It's some kind of throwback to our Neanderthal roots, how changes to our environment and the seasons brought fear and worry. When I think about this, I get it; change can be scary, especially change we didn't plan or want. Well, bloody hell, what's another name for menopause? Yes, ten points to you: THE CHANGE. Cue dramatic music.

As part of the changes, you might be having some brain fog moments in your life right now. I'm hoping you can have a good laugh at some of them. So far, my list has included:

1. attempting to cook chicken—without turning on the oven
2. forgetting the sugar when I made a birthday cake
3. putting the electric kettle on the gas burner to heat up the water
4. and leaving my wallet at home when I was grocery shopping for the week—not only did I have to leave everything at the checkout but I didn't have any money to get out of the parking lot.

Funny at the time? Perhaps not. But now, I can laugh at myself, as can the kids, and my husband . . . and my parents. Okay, so just about everyone is laughing at me. But at least we are laughing together. ☺

Is there a cure for brain fog? Certainly, getting a good night's sleep will be hugely helpful. Having a 20-minute nap does wonders for my brain, as does a 20-minute meditation, and of course all the usual good guys help, too: exercise, lots of water, and keeping stress levels way down.

Letter to my brain fog

Dear Brain Fog,

Sorry to bring this up again, but could you, for the love of GOD do something about your memory?

I don't know what, or how, but when you can't remember the name of your brother-in-law, whom you've known for 23 years, you scare me a little.

Oh, and shut down at night, okay? We all need a rest.

Love,
Me

Growth is uncomfortable because you've never been here before—you've never been this version of you. So give yourself a little grace and breathe through it.

Kristen Lohr
....

Pelvic floor

You know you are getting old when everything either dries up or leaks.

How can I not mention the weakened menopausal pelvic floor?

There is a new yoga move in my repertoire called, 'Bound-legged sneeze'. I've discovered this is of utmost importance as I've aged. You might be familiar with it yourself—it's the result of having a bowling ball sit inside your uterus, on top of your bladder, before being pushed out through a very small opening.

I loved being pregnant, and while there are many issues I needed to deal with while growing a baby, the weakened bladder is one that lingered longer than I realised. It was all fun and games while I was carrying a small human in my uterus. It all made perfect sense; people accepted the rush to the bathroom, the urinary jocularity: 'Don't make me laugh or I'll pee myself.'

It's a simple symptom of being pregnant. #adorable

Now that I've aged it's not so funny.

Now I can't bounce with my kids on the trampoline without feeling like I *am* going to pee myself.

I observed a situation a few years back with a friend of mine, who in her mid fifties and as a mother of two warned me of the need to take care with the dreaded pee escape.

We were having a birthday party for one of my children and we'd rented one of those bouncy blow-up castle things. Super fun. So when the kids all went home the adults who had been eyeing it all day moved in, as you do.

Hilarity ensued.

Laughter can be a bladder's worst enemy, but then add bouncing.

You know where I'm heading with this, right?

Well, before my friend could get out and go to the bathroom, it happened. The inevitable. We were getting paper towels and doing a little mop up.

It was only women around at the time. We understood.

Now I relate way more as I cross my legs to sneeze, and ditto for laughing. Jump rope seems to be a thing of the past, too.

I'll admit I have not been faithfully doing my Kegels, as suggested by a few. It's just not on my radar to remember to do ten minutes of flexing my pelvic floor. I'd rather have a cup of tea.

I did google 'pelvic floor assistance' out of interest. There are all sorts of apparatuses to improve yourself. Ready?

'The Kegelmaster'. Amazing. It's a whole machine, with springs and things, and comes with a log for your bladder habits. You know, like if she's been out late drinking with the girls, is more grouchy lately or staying in her room more often.

There are barbells to strengthen your vagina. Varbells? Barginas? Anyway, I'll let you use your imagination for that one.

And invented by Dr Kegel himself, the 'Perineometer', which tells you how fast your vagina can run. It also gives audio as well as visual biofeedback, so you can have a little chat with your vagina and encourage her to, 'grip a little harder please'.

Kegels. Ladies. Like the Nike ad recommends, 'Just do it'. But make sure you find out the correct way to do them.

I have no doubt women of ancient times were doing their own form of Kegels before it was named by a man.

All this did have me thinking that a good exercise routine might just do away with the cross-legged dance, and could get me back on the trampoline again.

I enrolled in a physio Pilates class and my teacher is awesome. She knows the ins and out of the pelvic floor like nobody's business. Standing there in a room full of women as we grip and release, I have hopes that one day I can laugh *and* bounce again.

It seems all it really takes is a little focus, commitment, and a thank you to my pelvic floor for hanging in there.

I do hope I've not offended anyone who suffers from incontinence on a permanent basis. I know it's a medical condition women and men suffer from. For me, ironically, it helps to laugh. As long as I cross my legs.

Let's talk vaginas

Vaginal dryness. There, I wrote it. Didn't want to, but it's there in black and white. When I read about this possible symptom of menopause I was horrified by the term 'vaginal atrophy'. There is a visual to those two words that left me feeling so anxious and scared. Thinking of any part of my body with the term 'atrophy' attached to it immediately makes me feel like some wrapped mummy from ancient Egypt.

So what is vaginal atrophy?

It's the thinning, drying and inflammation of the walls of your vagina. This happens due to the decline of oestrogen in our bodies. It's also one of the most under-reported symptoms we may experience, due to embarrassment. This particular symptom plays a huge part in why we may not want sex. Why would we when not only are we dealing with the physical discomfort but what we may be feeling emotionally around experiencing this symptom?

Feeling turned on without the lubrication that naturally occurred a year ago is confusing and alarming.

Do not despair!

Not all women experience this, some may experience different degrees of it, and there is assistance. Talking to a gynaecologist is helpful. There are oestrogen creams, suppositories, multiple lubes. I've added a list in the 'Help' chapter for natural lubes as well.

And while I wasn't exactly jumping for joy about this particular remedy, research shows that one of the best things you can do is keep having sex and/or masturbate.

This may go against everything you are feeling. If a part of your body is in pain, our natural instinct and usually the doctor's orders are to rest that part of your body, right?

Not so with our vaginas; it's like a muscle we need to keep exercising to keep lubricated so she can be fit and happy. Basically, like the rest of our bodies.

Seesaw symptoms

WAIT, I THOUGHT I WAS DONE?

Let's talk periods. As in, they are gone or going. I don't miss my cycle when it's gone for months at a time. There is a definite freedom in not having to calculate if my cycle will land on that beach holiday, or how bloated I'll be beforehand. The soaking of the sheets or underwear is now relegated to when my youngest has a nosebleed. Though, with that said, I miss my fertility.

Nine months of no menstrual cycle. Thinking that was it, my cycle was well and truly in the rear-view mirror, I handed over my pads and tampons to my daughters. And then I had my period. In hindsight, all the signs pointed towards my cycle beginning again: sore breasts, bloating, being super tired and more emotional. But those are also symptoms of perimenopause, so how could I know what was what?! When my cycle started again it was in full bloom like when I was a 30-year-old, which meant two things:

1. I was still in perimenopause.
2. I needed to begin the countdown again for menopause. (Remember it's at least one whole year without your cycle till you can say you are postmenopausal.)

Journal entry, May 2019

I can't keep up. I can't keep up with the decline of what my body is capable of doing. In relation to exercise and dieting, if I don't exercise for a week I look down and see bubbles of cellulite that have cascaded down to my ankles. Is it my imagination or is that really the truth? I don't even know anymore. I can't keep up. I can't keep up with the pain in my knees now or the new pain in my hip that is causing me to not be able to sit cross-legged. Is that it? Has that gone now? Will I never sit cross-legged again? What is that new pain? Why do my elbows hurt? What did I do? What's next? The neck is already an issue and has been for a while. Feel like I just can't keep up with the wall that is slowly but surely tumbling down, brick by brick, and I can't fix the hole in the wall fast enough.

Wrinkles should merely indicate where smiles have been.

Mark Twain
....

Journal entry, July 2019

Feeling like my symptoms have shifted again. Hot flushes are only a couple a day now. The weather has cooled so that's helping, thank God. It's the skin on my face now that's doing something new, it's crazy itchy. I feel sorry for my body. That's it's never been good enough, and meanwhile it's done everything I've asked it to. Continued breathing while I slept, grew humans perfectly. Healed wounds when I fell. To add to the itch on my face, my chest has now broken out in a rash. Hello, new symptom. I will be checking this one out with the doctor as it could be something other than perimenopause. The changes with my skin just keep rolling on: crepey, bumpy, dry and, of course, itchy.

Revolution has arrived

I have reached an age when, if someone tells me to wear socks, I don't have to.

Albert Einstein
....

I am a high school dropout. I mention this to a lot of people, apparently. My girlfriend told me the other day I told her this one fact four times over the first couple of hikes we did together. It's an attempt to offset any possible feeling that she might think I am better than her because I was a model, that I was held up as an image of pretty, so I make it clear that she is way smarter (which technically is true with this certain friend) and that I struggle with self-confidence, in the hope that will put her at ease, that she won't feel less beautiful in my presence somehow. Which is impossible as she is totally gorgeous in her own right.

Meanwhile, my girlfriend is thinking, why the hell does she keep repeating herself and why didn't I bring my water bottle? She didn't give a rat's arse, it just comes down to the crap cycling around my head. I've done this multiple times with multiple women; I concede my wisdom or smarts so they feel more comfortable. All the while they are *not* feeling uncomfortable about anything . . . it's just me when my ex-model brain kicks in.

I realised I made an unconscious agreement that I'm now making sure I am undoing. I could be pretty but not smart— pretty might be threatening to other women, so best to dumb yourself down, best to keep small.

We need to give girls and women permission to be anything and everything. Actually, strike that. Who said there is even the need for permission? Permission from whom? We can just simply *be* all that we can and want to be.

I realise that I have been systematically hiding from myself in large and small ways for the past 30-odd years.

I remember sitting in my house in Los Angeles after I had concluded the usual round of dropping off one child, carpooling another, and picking up groceries for dinner—a routine I was very comfortable with, and yet a routine that had been the same for a long time. Yes, I have worked different jobs and loved them, though until that simple moment of sitting at home and thinking, 'Is this it?' everything was feeling like *Groundhog Day*. Everything felt safe—I knew what lay ahead, what the needs of my family and the household was—but I wanted more. I wasn't sure what the more was, I just knew I felt restless.

Since moving to Australia and turning my life upside down at the same time as experiencing perimenopause, I've felt I've been pushed to change so many things. Yes, I've chosen to change, and actually it's not so much a *change* rather than a reveal. What's been fluttering inside me for so long finally has broken free.

In some ways I feel like I didn't have any other choice but to reveal myself.

In order to not be steamrolled by menopause, I had to make friends with not only my symptoms but my entire new and ever-changing body. I had to hold menopause's hand and say, 'Okay, we are going through this together. I will deal with each symptom as it arises. I will make the best of this time and love myself through this.'

Women do get through this time, somehow or another, and often at the end they think, 'Hey, look at me now', or 'Look at who I have become'.

We can change our outlook and priorities and focus on the health of our bodies and minds and the health of our families and relationships. We can have it all. It can all be the precursor to living our lives in a real, positive way.

Change also means revolution. I love that—that menopause is a revolution for the mind and body.

As I stand with hands on my ever-widening hips, with my feet grounded and my stance wide, ready and facing the next step in my life, the wind not only in my hair but blowing my extra chin hairs about, I think: I need a cup of tea, my back aches and I need to sit down and get the hell off my feet.

What I also think is: we have limited days left here on this earth, in this body, so why waste them hating ourselves, hating our bodies, our lives?

Sometimes I'm overwhelmed with all the 'have tos' in this world. You 'have to' work out, eat healthy, love your body, look good, take care of yourself, engage with people, eat, drink loads of water, feed your kids (okay, that should not be a 'have to'). They can start to feel like pressure. I don't do well under pressure, especially pressure from the outside. Pressure to look a certain way, act and perform in a certain way. So that can leave me some-where in the middle, swinging between what I 'have to', 'want to' or 'need to' do. When I find my way to 'want to', not only am I making a change just for myself, but everything becomes connected to the desires of my heart.

Letter to mirrors at clothing stores

Dear Mirrors at Clothing Stores,

Ahh, look. I know you're doing your job, reflecting back what I'm trying on, but for the LOVE OF GOD can you do something about the lighting in the change rooms? Never do I feel uglier than when I try on clothes in a store. I'm fairly certain there is a large pool of women that would agree with me. That one of you that shows what I look like from behind . . . it haunts me. So, softer lighting, a gentle voice-over telling us all to 'love our shape' or that we're 'so much more than that bikini' we are trying on. Just an idea.

Love,
Me

Nothing ages as poorly as a beautiful woman's ego.[1]

Paulina Porizkova
....

Aging

Aging is not lost youth but a new stage of opportunity and strength.

Betty Friedan
....

I'm driving in the car with my family. I'm in the passenger seat. It's summer and my arm is resting on the open window. I can see my reflection in the side mirror. My spaghetti strap dress is blowing in the breeze. What is also somewhat blowing and most definitely jiggling is the extra flesh that has accumulated on my arms. I've never seen this on my body in the light of day. I'm kind of fascinated. I grab and squeeze, shake and wobble.

I flash to a memory: it's my nanna cooking in her kitchen, and I see those same arms, wobbling away as she chops the potatoes for dinner.

Nanna arms. They have arrived.

For so long my arms have been slim and fairly taut, so this new scenario is fresh, even if I don't feel fresh looking them. I had been so used to getting away with minimal exercise to stay the same size, minimal exercise to keep sagging body parts at bay. But here I was, aging, with everything heading south.

It's a weird experience to feel young in my brain but see a 51-year-old woman in the mirror.

Fear of aging is a well-worn path. I understand that with the changes we all go through, the march towards our demise is often what scares us the most.

What will we look like when we age, when we hit 60, 70, 80? And if we have defined ourselves by our looks and they fade, or change, who are we?

I didn't grow up thinking much about my looks at all. Around the age of fifteen, sixteen I started being noticed for my appearance. I don't remember being complimented on my intelligence or my ability to read well or anything outside of what I looked like once I hit fifteen. I was gaining attention and praise for something, and that something was my external appearance. This set me up for all sorts of issues in the future, I just didn't know it yet. I didn't have to work for my 'pretty'. There was no degree of hard labour involved. It was simply the right mix of good genes. And those good genes opened doors for me. Those doors were wonderful, they led to a modelling career that I'm proud of, though my modelling career is far and away not the total sum of my life. It's the most memorable aspect of me for other people, and the most shiny. It was definitely the most well paid!

> If beauty is your calling card that will start to fade, that is a challenge because what happens when what you look like begins to change?
>
> *Oprah Winfrey*
> ....

People treat people differently when they are beautiful; it's a fact of human nature. I needed to settle into understanding who I was without the modelling. That of course didn't begin for me until I left the modelling industry and ploughed headlong into careers that were as far from modelling as possible. Eventually those genes that served me well as a young woman who was booked for the covers of magazines changed, and the gift of pretty started to look different.

Sure, I was still an attractive 30- and 40-year-old, though that youthful glow, as they say, was fading. I remember walking down a street in Los Angeles with my eldest daughter, watching her cut a swathe through the crowd, and, unbeknownst to her, having many a young and older man turn their heads to check her out. I also remember this being me when I was her age; I was always uncomfortable with that attention, always. Watching these men and the effect that my daughter had on them made me feel incredibly protective of her, and realising I was no longer the one who turned heads made me realise I was definitely aging.

It was freeing to not be recognised when I moved to Los Angeles and began other careers. I was out from under the label of 'model'. Every so often I would be approached by someone and asked if I ever thought about trying to be a model.

Who me? Nah.

I feel fortunate, because I chose to leave the fashion industry. It wasn't that I was no longer wanted. I wasn't pushed out because I had aged, even though there is always another round of models coming up behind you with better cheekbones or longer legs. But the definition of my real beauty changed for me when I left the industry. If I had not done the inner work and found careers that fulfilled my heart and soul, I would've been in real trouble.

I love the road my life has taken since leaving the modelling industry. I feel proud of the work I did and still do with children, and supporting women through birth. I've loved it all.

The irony is not lost on me that here I am as an over-50-year-old and lamenting that women my age are not represented in the media enough. Meanwhile, 30 years ago I never gave a thought to what 50-year-old women might have thought as I posed in front of a camera advertising skin care or clothes.

Unconsciously I was part of the beauty myth: that beautiful is better, that young girls wanted to be me, look like me. That somehow I was the idea of the 'perfect woman'. Even more than that—the true-blue Aussie gal. Actually, my heritage is Danish and Irish, there's not an Indigenous bone in my body, and I felt far from perfect.

It saddens me to think that my looks were held up as the ideal, when there were plenty of brown-skinned, dark-haired little girls who did not see their reflection looking back at them from magazine covers.

So my relationship with beauty is a complicated one. One that I'm finding menopause is assisting me to understand.

We tend to hold on to what we once were in order to maintain value in our lives. Sometimes that value is how beautiful we were. I had to cultivate my inner world, because external things always fade away. I'm learning through menopause to not be attached to the external version of myself. To not be defined by what other people think of how I look. That as a woman who once made a career out of being pretty, I now have a strong voice made from my life experiences.

Aging has allowed me to focus on myself more than ever, and that's a good thing. My health is becoming a big priority.

My dear dad has a saying whenever he forgets something or has his seventh doctor's visit in a month . . . he tells me to, 'not get old, darling'. My response is always, 'It's better than the alternative, Dad.'

The bottom line is that it's a gift to even be in a position to age. I lament and moan at times, curse and eyeroll, but being alive is a privilege.

I'm baffled that anyone might not think women get more beautiful as they get older. Confidence comes with age, and looking beautiful comes from the confidence someone has in themselves.

Kate Winslet
....

I've been working on speaking my truth and my feelings honestly for so long now, from the young girl who felt so insecure, to the teenage model who allowed herself to be pushed and pulled, and the young wife and mother who subdued her anger and was so afraid to upset anyone. Aging and menopause have made me softer and stronger. I see the changes in my body, I see the soft belly and arms, the jowls that sit a little lower, the droopier eyelids, and I also feel the strength of my wisdom and my voice. I love my mother's face, and I see my face changing to reflect hers—how can I love her face but not my own?

In an article from *Counseling Today* titled 'Falling Short of Perfect', Laurie Meyers quotes counsellor Laura Hensley Choate, who describes how 'Women throughout history have been valued "only for their beauty and fertility".' She also says, 'Although these qualities are no longer the sole source of a woman's worth, youth and beauty are still most valued.'[2]

This is where menopause can throw a spanner in the works. Because, as it stands, once a woman ages those qualities may diminish and by society's standards she loses value.

No. Way.

All of my friends and most of the women I know are in some stage of menopause, either peri or post, and my God they have so much value! We all have so much knowledge, so much that those around us can learn from, and yet held up to what society says is valuable, we somehow fall short because we have aged.

Hence, we have a booming plastic surgery industry. Never have Botox, fillers, facelifts and body-altering surgeries been more popular. The pressure tends to be greater on women as in general most men do not feel the same compulsion to appear young.

So from the get-go we are in a disadvantaged position. When I see women who have had a facelift or Botox, I understand. I do not for a second judge any woman who has felt the need to snip here or get a lift there, because we've been fed an abnormal idea of beauty and aging simply by being born female. And looking after yourself physically, through whatever means, is important. I'm a big believer in doing whatever makes you feel better about yourself, but I want the feeling to come from inside, not from feeling that you have to live up to some unreachable standard. The message from the media is that a woman's primary value is sex, which equals physical attractiveness.

Menopause is our opportunity to step off into freedom.

We may act sophisticated and worldly but I believe we feel safest when we go inside ourselves and find home, a place where we belong and maybe the only place we really do.

Maya Angelou
....

Letter to my bum

Dear Bum,

Girl, you got big and sweaty. Are you planning on staying that size? I mean, it's fine, it's just that my pants really need to know. They are confused as hell. Also, if you could stop eating my underwear I'd really appreciate it. Reminder to you from the late great Freddie Mercury, when he sung about how, 'Fat-bottomed girls make the rockin' world go round'.

Love,
Me

Our thoughts are the most important makeup we wear each day, and this is a friendly reminder to see and appreciate the entirety of your beauty as often as you can.

Light Watkins
....

Body-mind and menopause

Symptoms are our body's way of saying that our bodies are out of balance and need healing. For years I studied and taught the body–mind connection with Doreen Rivera in Los Angeles. Body–mind work is a lot like being a detective, an archaeologist, a mapmaker and a historian (of yourself) all rolled into one. Knowledge is power, and understanding the physical body and the way it relates to your emotions is empowering.

I would teach an exercise class that looked similar to a cross between yoga and floor Pilates. The classes have been an integral part of my healing. My body has never let me down in offering up information—sometimes I haven't wanted to take a look at the information arising, but inevitably I know I can't run from my body, because 'the body does not lie'. I could try to hide emotionally, but my body always tells the story, either by breaking down, or stiffening up—sending me a signal.

Learning about body–mind has been like having the most informative friend with me 24 hours a day; it's just a matter of listening. In class we would have a journal by our side to record any feelings or thoughts that might arise as we moved through the exercises. As Doreen would say, 'When you move muscle you move emotion.' Emotions are stored in our cells, including any traumas from childhood, whether they be physical or emotional. In fact, any kind of trauma, at any age, the body remembers. And without releasing the emotions and healing what has been left unhealed, our bodies can become 'dis-eased'. When we feel sad or depressed, anxious or angry we often have physical signals that go along with the mental and emotional anguish. Stress will bring a headache on faster than anything.

Specific body parts correspond to where we hold emotions. The lungs are primarily grief; the liver, anger; our shoulders and neck are responsibility; the lower back is how we support ourselves; the feet, our foundation.

So where does menopause fit into all this?

When I think about the symptoms that menopause is connected to and the emotional aspects of those symptoms, what is revealed is how important this time is for women. How much our bodies are talking to us.

For myself, my breasts have grown bigger—breasts are how we nurture babies; breasts in themselves represent nurturance. I am being called to nurture myself at this time. As I've mentioned before, this is an ongoing theme for me. I've been the nurturer for so long of others and I'm truly learning now what it means to nurture myself.

Our uterus and ovaries are where we create life, so as they call our attention the question is, 'What are we going to create *now*?'

Our bellies are the 'belly of emotion', the all-important place where we hold our unspoken feelings, especially our deep emotional expressions. You know the sayings, 'I felt like I was hit in the guts when I heard that', or 'My belly had butterflies', or 'My belly was so tense because of how scared I was'. Often children have a bellyache when they are distressed but can't or don't want to put words to what they are feeling. So as my belly has expanded, perhaps the signal is, 'What emotions am I holding on to?' 'What feeling do I need to speak to, rather than hold inside?'

Joint pain? Well, joints are the literal articulation of movement of one part of the body connected to another. I have joint pain in my elbows. The arms are about embracing; what am I not embracing? What am I telling myself about my ability to embrace myself? Especially at this time of my life?

Just those questions alone are helpful in getting me to look at my life and its intricacies. They form a breadcrumb trail that leads me back to my heart and everything connected to it—how I want to love who I am, exactly as I am. How I want to applaud myself for all that I have done in my life.

Knees are also another articulation point. The bending of the knees is what allows us to take steps forward—we cannot progress forward well unless we bend our knees. Knees can represent the fear of moving forward. There is a lot of fear around menopause and what's happening to my body, what's coming next. Will my memory be affected? My sex life? My relationships? How I look? Plus that fear of aging in general. So does it not make sense that the knee pain coinciding with menopause means that in this new phase of life there can be fear involved?

Letter to my eyebrows

Dear Eyebrows,

Did I offend you in some way? I'm so sorry if the plucking somehow hurt your feelings. I see you've decided to migrate south onto my chin. That's fine, I guess. I don't want to come across as, well, anti-chin hairs. I'm far from it. I just liked you better when you were back above my eyes. Filling in the gaps that are now being filled in with a pencil. You are welcome back anytime, no questions asked. It's really not all that fun on my chin by the way. It only takes one good look in the car mirror with some tweezers and you are history. Sorry. Come on home.

Love,
Me

Letter to my cellulite

Dear Cellulite,

Fuck off.

Love,
Me

I will hold this body tender after years too many spent callously rending it apart. I will stroke this skin with adulation, forever cherishing the braille tales of survival it has to tell and to myself I will speak gentle words of adoration instead of letting the venom of loathe drip forth from my lips. My body is uniquely mine to love and cherish and I will no longer let it be my battleground.

Becca Lee
....

What's your vagina's name?

First letter of your first name.	First letter of your last name.
A. Princess	A. Hot Waffle
B. Cuddly	B. Glitter Biscuit
C. Empress	C. Lunchbox
D. Wonderful	D. Love Muffin
E. Dainty	E. Sugar Hole
F. Mrs	F. Wonder Bush
G. The Glorious	G. Thunder Bush
H. The Incredible	H. Chomp Box
I. President	I. Muff
J. The Magnificent	J. Jiggly Bits
K. Lady	K. Love Button
L. The Insatiable	L. Thunder Dungeon
M. The Talented	M. Love Bunker
N. Fancy	N. Destroyer
O. Sparkly	O. Danger Bin
P. The Bald	P. Whisker Biscuit
Q. The Tiny	Q. Pearl Crusher
R. Mc	R. Crazy Beaver
S. Queen	S. Penis Glove
T. Madame	T. Banana Basket
U. Mega	U. Fuzz Box
V. Adorable	V. Pink Panther
W. Wild	W. Penis Fly Trap
X. The Reckless	X. Magical Land
Y. Fluffy	Y. Love Monster
Z. Mademoiselle	Z. Snake Charmer

@scary mommy
....

Just call me Princess Love Muffin from now on, okay?

Oh my God, what if you wake up some day, and you're 65, or 75, and you never got your memoir or novel written; or you didn't go swimming in warm pools and oceans all those years because your thighs were jiggly and you had a nice big comfortable tummy; or you were just so strung out on perfectionism and people-pleasing that you forgot to have a big juicy creative life, of imagination and radical silliness and staring off into space like when you were a kid? It's going to break your heart. Don't let this happen.

Anne Lamott

CHAPTER 7

Myths of menopause

I wish I could show you, when you are lonely or in darkness,
the astonishing light of your own being.

HAFIZ

Myth 1: There's something wrong with you

There is nothing 'wrong' with menopause. It's as natural a part of life as puberty. Changes may happen, yes. But it's not an illness. Our bodies may feel like they are telling us something different, but if I use a different language than 'something is wrong with me', then I can assist myself in staying curious about what *is* happening and how best I can support myself. In this time in our lives great things can happen: a new worldview, a change in career. Focus on changing the negative into a positive. Holding this ideal is a fight against the lies women have been told since day one. We need to do it for the next generation of women coming behind us.

My mission, should I choose to accept it, is to find peace
with exactly who and what I am. To take pride in my
thoughts and appearance, my talents, my flaws and to stop
this incessant worrying that I can't be loved as I am.

Anais Nin
....

Myth 2: Your health will deteriorate

Currently I'm the healthiest I've been in many years. This has
been my greatest positive from menopause. I've figured out which
foods work for me and which ones don't. I've taken up yoga and
Pilates. I make sure I move my body some way or another every
day. Am I heavier than I was in my thirties? Sure, and I am
learning to accept my new body shape. But I am healthier by far
now than I was back then! I'm taking greater care with many
aspects of my health. Regular check-ups with my naturopath,
upping my intake of vitamins and minerals. And healthier eating.
When you feel better, you live longer.

Myth 3: You are no longer attractive

What? A woman owning who she is, not feeling the pressure
to compete with other women is not only attractive but freeing.
True beauty comes from within. A woman at peace with herself is
magical. That takes time to learn, so the age we are when we enter
menopause is about the age when we understand this better than

ever. And that's a beautiful thing. This may have come naturally to you—perhaps you already had a wonderful sense of yourself and the beauty that is *you*. I applaud you, woman! I'm still working on this. Menopause didn't make me ugly; I already felt ugly many times throughout my life. What menopause is doing for me is making me go, 'Honey, it's so *not* about how you look, it's about how you feel and owning yourself as a wise woman.' Not only is that a gift I gain from menopause, it's a lifelong challenge that I finally feel I'm embracing.

> And the beauty of a woman, with passing years only grows.
>
> *Audrey Hepburn*
> ....

Myth 4: Natural remedies don't work

Hormone replacement therapy (HRT) is the standard treatment for menopause that is available to many women. But consider also the option of complementary medicine. Most of my friends travelled through menopause resorting only to natural remedies, and I have found relief from them myself. Be aware that just because a medicine is 'natural' doesn't mean that it is without side effects or risks, but there are natural treatments that have been shown to be effective with minimal or no side effects. Be sure to discuss treatment options—mainstream or complementary—with your doctor first.

Everyone's body is different; some medicines, herbal or not, will work for some and not for others. I had to change my remedies periodically as my body seemed to get used to one remedy and the symptoms would come back. Keeping track of my symptoms helped me enormously. Why not give different naturopathic modalities a go? There are so many great healers and treatments available out there: Reiki, biofeedback, visualisation and guided imagery, homeopathy, Chinese medicine, dancing naked in the rain. Just to name a few. You might be surprised and find someone to assist you who knows exactly what you and your body need.

Myth 5: Menopause causes depression for everyone

It would be easy to say this, especially for those of us who have experienced depression in our perimenopausal years. According to studies, women are twice as likely to experience depression than men.[1]

Changes in the hormones oestrogen and progesterone, like when we have experienced PMS, can be responsible for mood swings. But going through menopause does not mean you will *automatically* feel depressed or have any mood swings. Some conditions might put women at a higher risk of depression—they could be a history of depression, poor physical health and high levels of stress. Handling the changes in our bodies and fertility can be daunting, sure, but we've handled way more than that in our lifetime! Menopause can be a time where emotions become unearthed, and feelings that have been long suppressed come to the surface. This may also feel overwhelming, so getting the support you need will not only be beneficial to your health, it can help make this a positive, life-changing time.

Myth 6: Menopause is the reason for weight gain

Our metabolism slows down between the ages of 35 and 55, so that extra weight around our tummies and thighs, well, it was kind of heading our way anyway! I know plenty of women who did not gain any weight during their perimenopause/menopause changes. It does mean it's important to be aware of what we eat and exercise regularly. (I did neither of these things . . . hello weight gain.) Sleeping well is key for me; the less I sleep, the more I gain weight. It's the way my body works.

> A beautiful face will age and a perfect body will change, but a beautiful soul will always be a beautiful soul.
>
> *Author unknown*
> ....

Myth 7: Your sex life is ruined by menopause

Ruined? No. Changed? Possibly. You might need to invest in some lubricants. Many women actually feel a sense of freedom with the knowledge there is no risk of pregnancy. Other women experience a rise in testosterone, which might make you have 'throwing down your partner in the middle of the day with the curtains open'-type sex. Menopause is not a death sentence to your sex life. You and your partner might need to have some serious talks about how to be intimate in a different way than you were before. Just *having* that conversation can be the start of a new level of intimacy that you may have never realised was possible.

Myth 8: Menopause begins at 50

There is no magic number for menopause. I have a friend who started when she was 35, as did all the women in her family. I also know of another woman who was still having her monthly cycle at 56! Again, it will be different for every woman. Most commonly, menopause begins around the 45 to 55 age range.

Myth 9: Hot flushes are the first sign of menopause

The first sign for me was my irregular periods, followed by fatigue and sleep issues. Hot flushes are a common symptom of menopause but don't signify the onset of menopause. You might find, looking back, there were other symptoms that began earlier. Cravings, anxiety, breast tenderness or brain fog were perhaps the beginning for some women.

Myth 10: Menopause symptoms are severe for all women

Okay, now let's all breathe a deep sigh of relief here. I know women who had barely a rise in temperature or a grouchy moment during menopause. It can be said that those of us whose symptoms tend to be more severe will be more vocal about it. Because, quite frankly, I need to be vocal about what I'm feeling or I'll totally combust. Others interpret their sensations in a way that is all-out positive. Those women are surviving the apocalypse and need a medal.

It's very easy to read negative information about menopause, and the more I researched the darker the news became. And my thought was, 'Holy Crap, I might not even *survive* menopause.' Yet I've *not* experienced many of the symptoms that have been lobbed about in the media and that I've found through google searches. You do you.

Certain studies have found that up to 80 per cent of women experiencing menopause report no decrease in quality of life and only about 10 percent report feelings of despair, irritability or fatigue during the menopause transition.[2]

Dr Axe
....

Myth 11: Menopause causes global warming

Little known fact, menopause is *not* the cause of climate change. Yes, you might be experiencing a tropical world under your sheets at night, but the heat you're emitting will not melt the poles. In fact, you are trained and ready for any rise in global temperatures thanks to your menopause. Could you survive in the Gobi Desert? Yes. Live in Death Valley? No worries. Trek through the heart of the Simpson Desert mid-summer with ease. You are a hot flush warrior able to thrive and survive in extreme heat at any point in the day or night. You win.

And once the storm is over you won't remember how you made it through, how you managed to survive. You won't even be sure, in fact, whether the storm is really over. But one thing is certain. When you come out of the storm you won't be the same person who walked in. That's what this storm's all about.

Haruki Murakami, Kafka on the Shore

CHAPTER 8

Her story, his story, your story

When we share our stories, we open our hearts to allow
others to share their stories. It gives us all the sense that we
are not alone on this journey.[1]

JANINE SHEPHERD

In an *Everyday Health* article[2] an interesting connection between
culture and menopause is made. The author, Eric Berlin MD,
writes of how Western women have a different perspective on
not only their place in this world, but also comparisons to each
other, our thoughts on growing old and the value of wisdom of
the older generations.

Berlin's article goes on to explain that Mayan Indian women:

reported no hot flushes or any significant menopausal
symptoms. Mayan women tend to look forward to menopause

because with it comes a progressive change in status within their communities and, in turn, a feeling of freedom. When women from indigenous cultures cross into menopause, they often become known as 'wise women' or spiritual leaders and hold a place of power in their communities.[3]

Curiously I've read about how symptoms manifest themselves differently in different cultures. Asian women report much lower rates of menopause-related symptoms than Western women. Why? This is possibly linked to diet, but prevailing thought suggests that it may be the result of Asian attitudes towards aging. The Japanese word for this phase in our lives is *konenki*, which translates to 'renewal years' and 'energy'.

So if Western women changed their outlook and views on menopause, could we actually be proud of the phase we are in? Would our symptoms be more like a badge of honour? How would our symptoms change for us if we welcomed them?

I'm always amazed at the ability of women to go deep quickly. Even with women I've only just met, the conversation can turn personal at the speed of light. Before I know it, I'm discussing miscarriages, aggravating husbands, raging thoughts and lack of sleep. We magnetise, like an organism, then we multiply—our thoughts, our energy—and share the mood, the pain, the laughs and the healing. Whenever I've talked about my experiences with other women I feel the relief of sharing and connecting. In relating to each other, we can ease the burden of what we are feeling. Magic.

When I first started researching menopause online for assistance I couldn't find anything, really, that helped with my emotional wellbeing. I read plenty about how I would most likely have mood swings, or possibly depressive thoughts. There sure is an enormous amount of information about all the negative symptoms you might experience with menopause; there were days when I was doing research for this book that I couldn't believe how much bad press is given to this time in our lives. But there was nothing to help *prepare* me for a downswing of feelings. I needed something tangible I could use when I was at the bottom of the pit. Once I was there, I couldn't reach out, so to have something I could read or listen to may have given me the lifeline to grab hold off. What I needed was stories that helped me to feel I was not alone in my experiences. That other women before me had been through menopause, that women also found *benefits* to menopause, and that some women had sailed through menopause with nary a symptom.

I've been surprised by everything relating to menopause: how intense the hot flushes are, how deep into depression I fell, how angry I felt. And now that I'm seeing a light at the end of the tunnel, I'm surprised at the feeling of renewal.

Someone to listen to us, to hear us, to relate to what we are talking about, especially when we are in pain, be it emotional or physical, can be the difference between depression and healing. When someone utters the magical words, 'I know exactly what you mean', there's an internal sigh of relief that I am not alone in feeling crazy, hurt, fat, sad, at a loss at what to do. I would have loved for the older women in my life to sit me down and say, 'Okay, here we go, let me fill you in on some things you may feel'. Some of my friends just kept so quiet about their menopause, my only clue would be a fanning of their faces when they broke out in a sweat.

> I know people heal by being able to tell the story—the whole story.
>
> *Clarissa Pinkola Estés*
> ....

Let's tell our stories in safe places, tell them so you can hear them out loud and be heard as well. Tell them for the next woman that might need a boost or some information. Following are some generous women who have agreed to talk a little about their menopause experience. I'm so grateful to them for sharing their intimate feelings for you to read.

Traci's story

I was 47 when I started menopause. I really didn't know much about it. My mum, sister and grandma all had hysterectomies so I had no history to go off.

My periods were hell. I started my cycle at fourteen and, for over 30 years, every month I was laid out for seven days. The doctors finally figured out I was anaemic.

PMS was awful. I was either suicidal, homicidal or depressed.

When menopause happened my cycle just simply stopped. It was very gentle. I had some hot flushes, but I wasn't having the same ups and downs as I did when I had my cycle. I feel more even now.

What's changed is that a bit of my brain chemistry feels different. My memory is not as good, though I feel like I could fix that if I ate better.

My advice to women about to go through or going through menopause would be to breathe, give yourself a break, acknowledge that this is part of the cycle of life. It's a great thing, full of new opportunities—your energy levels change for the better.

When I went through menopause, having children was completely off the table, so even though I was never compelled to be a mother, having that off the table was like . . . Yes! That's not even part of the conversation now. So breathe, acknowledge, take the time to be quiet with yourself.

My advice to partners is to be kind, communicate, ask questions, be considerate. I grew up in an era when your period was something to be denigrated. Honour the women in your life and be patient.

Anita's story

I was around 47 when I started perimenopause

My menstrual cycle was very, very heavy for five days followed by two okay days. I felt like I had a tummy problem. The week before, too.

The most challenging part of menopause has been the sudden sadness, the emotional rollercoaster: crying easily, sobbing at times, as I felt my old life was gone and I no longer felt like me! I never felt good. I worked full time, exercised when I could, went to yoga and relaxed as much as possible when I was not working or else I could not cope.

I am a very private person in some ways and felt I could not talk to anyone about it as everyone seemed okay. I just felt like my mind was racing and my body could not keep up.

I had a hollow sadness in me and could not shake it. Loud music made me crazy for a long time.

I started to spend more time alone and just with my family. I did not feel the urge to be too social. Just content with peaceful-ness and quietness.

Now, looking back, I see the way I've changed for the better. I've become much more tolerant of people as I understood that people go through ups and downs all the time. Not just always up! I am married to a person who is always up and he could not understand and chose to pretend it was not any different. He did not like to talk about it as he did not like me being too emotional.

I have a daughter and if I was to give her or any woman about to go through menopause any advice, it would be to listen to your body and your mind. If it says no, then listen. Don't just do or say things because you want to be nice and happy. Let your feelings out and find someone who understands. Talk to your mother, sisters, friends and doctor. It's okay to know you feel different, and you are not going crazy but becoming more tolerant and less on-the-go all the time, and it's okay to do less of things you don't want to do and have more of the quiet and peacefulness.

Yoga, meditation, sleep, massage, acupuncture, long walks are all so good for you during this time.

Listen to what your body is telling you.

Would I do anything different in preparing myself for menopause? I had talked with my mum and she had started menopause about the same age. She did not remember feeling as fragile as I did but maybe things were different then. She also reminded me that she became a grandmother about the same age when my niece Lara was born and my mum and dad were so in love with her! It completely took over their lives!

My advice to the partners of women in menopause would be to listen, to be patient and to not try and pretend it's not a problem. To be supportive even more. And let me know that I'm not fat because I eat a lot but because my body changed with menopause.

And I said to my body, softly, 'I want to be your friend.' It took a long breath and replied, 'I have been waiting my whole life for this.'

Nayyirah Waheed
....

Maria's story

So I realised at 45 . . . all of a sudden I'd had no period for the month of December. The thoughts that followed . . . they were very dark. Pregnancy? My cycle, up until that point, had been very regular. However, the flow was different each month.

When I realised my body was changing—even though I'm not officially in menopause yet; I still have my period, whenever it shows up!—initially I felt old. Am I that old already? The cultural thing about menopause related to old age was engraved in me.

I'm not concerned about menopause. I'm open, with no expectations, and I look forward to not having any thoughts or worries about pregnancy!

I've changed, throughout the last few years. I'm very accepting of what is, and I've let go of many cultural things related to beauty (I stopped dying my hair and have a sleek short haircut). Weight . . . those extra pounds . . . oh well! And I've let go of feeling I need to be perfect, basically! Do I have a belly? What? My hip hurts. What?

I have two amazing daughters. My advice to them when they are embarking on their own menopause journey would be to take the right supplements, to use essential oils to reduce symptoms and my face cream, 'Egyptian magic', as a lubricant, and to educate their husbands/partners with patience to care for them! And enjoy sex! It's not all over yet!

If I could go back and prepare myself, I would like to un-listen to all the bad comments I ever heard about it and move on with ease. It can also have a good side! No more bloody pants, or pads!

My advice to partners is lubricate, make sure that she has a good time, give her a massage as often as you can! Kiss her good morning and goodnight with no judgement of how tired she is. Help her before she asks. Basically, read her thoughts!

I am appalled that the term we use to talk about aging is 'anti'. Aging is as natural as a baby's softness and scent. Aging is human evolution in its pure form.[4]

Jamie Lee Curtis
....

Neeyah's story

I started perimenopause somewhere around 48 to 50.

My cycle was always infrequent and spotty throughout my life; when I was in perimenopause my hot flushes were so much worse than when I reached menopause.

The best thing about going through menopause was realising I would no longer be having my monthly moon. I did have emotions around not ever having children, though I have so many children now around me. It was a very poignant time.

I became more serious, focused and determined to modify my diet because I wanted for the rest of my life to maintain a healthy optimal lifestyle. I really looked at what I was eating once I hit menopause.

My advice to women would be to cut back on sugar! I know for me sugar definitely contributed to hot flushes and mood swings and feeling depressed.

My advice for partners would be to be compassionate, loving and kind. This transformation is real. Be patient. Remember why you married her! Because you love her.

Louise's story

I always had the most painful periods. I had lots of days off school when I was young. At seventeen I was put on the pill because of it. Most months it felt like I was in first-stage labour. I had no reprieve after children. In fact, it just got worse.

It wasn't until I returned to Australia that I was diagnosed with endometriosis. My gynaecologist was amazed that I was able to have children . . . My husband's sperm count was (thankfully) incredibly high. Which, as you can imagine, he has worn with lots of pride.

After Sammy was born my periods were still very painful so I had a procedure and at the same time a Mirena IUD was inserted. This was okay for a while but it wasn't long before it was making me feel dreadful. I was never really well on the pill either. So I had the Mirena removed. The doctor thought I was making it up. But I felt instant relief when it was out . . . A woman knows her body.

Shortly after the Mirena was removed I started having perimenopause symptoms. I was pretty young, early-to-mid-forties. I had a blood test, but it didn't show anything. I have since been told that it is quite normal for a blood test not to show anything. It can depend on the time of your cycle as to when you have a blood test. My doctor didn't explain this. She didn't believe me when I asked for a blood test because I thought I was perimenopausal.

It was awful not to be believed. Not many women I knew were going through the same thing. I read a lot about it. I started talking to older women. I started exercising a lot more. I also started to take a lot of different vitamins. By talking and reading I discovered that by taking the strongest vitamin B supplement with the strongest magnesium supplement worked wonders. I started drinking herbal teas, too, especially at night.

Night-times were the most annoying as it was then that my bones would feel like they were on fire. Like burning rods of steel in my skin. My sleep was broken because I was so bloody hot. My husband would touch me and recoil saying, 'My God, you are hot.' Also, I can be in the deepest sleep and just wake up . . . and then be awake for hours, for no reason. So exhausting.

While I am talking about symptoms, I will also say that when I was right in the height of it I would feel so anxious. I am not usually like that. The vitamin B and magnesium were very helpful for this, too. It was a stressful time in our lives. My husband had lost his job and my son was struggling emotionally after his illness when he was thirteen. It was hard for me to decipher what was causing the feelings. I would also go crazy mad. This is something I really hated about myself. I also had no sex drive.

By 48 my periods had stopped. Coincidently both my sisters' and our mother's periods ended at the same age.

When my periods ended I did think 'fantastic, everything will go back to normal' . . . but *no*. It just goes on and on! What is that?!

I think I am slowly coming to the end of it. I still sometimes get hot at night. I am a lot more rational now and hopefully not as emotional. I want to always be fit and strong. I want to always be moving. I still don't have a strong sex drive. I think the experience has made me kinder and more patient. I don't care about things as much and I understand that time is movement and fluid, therefore nothing stays the same.

Partners of menopausal women need to be patient. They need to understand that they do not need to find a solution but just accept what is happening. To understand that at times their partner will think they are really going crazy. To know that their partner can cry, scream and be irrational but that they should not be offended. The partner of a menopausal woman should remain calm and rational. They need to know that it will pass. They need to understand that sometimes the woman won't be able to explain how she is feeling and that it's okay for them to want time alone.

My daughter unfortunately has inherited my inability to take the pill and also suffers badly from period pain. She will probably start menopause at the same age that I did. Fortunately, these things are spoken of much more readily now. We are already laughing about the hot flushes. She is already asking me questions. I just want her to know that I will be here for all her questions . . . and show her sympathy.

On New Year's Eve we were with close friends for dinner. My girlfriend began talking to me about how she was really struggling with menopause. She was a friend who had always said she was breezing through it. To be honest, I had been worried about her for a while. Her mother has serious mental health issues and she said it was that which made her insist that she was going to breeze through it. I was so pleased when she said that she was going to take action.

But this made me think. Often at this time in our lives we are going through changes with partners, family, work and aging parents. Often it is hard to decipher what is causing what. It is difficult to know if your child's anxiety is making you wake in the night or if your husband's job (or lack of) is making your stomach churn as school fees and mortgages need to be paid. The hot flushes are easily explainable, but so many of the symptoms are hard to categorise as one thing or another.

Pilates, walking and now yoga are my definite saviours. Luckily, I love my husband and of course my kids. Financially we are stable, and I have some beautiful friends. Life is thankfully on an even keel. Is this why my symptoms have reduced? I don't know the answer. But I will continue to take my vitamin B and magnesium. I will also continue to exercise and drink my herbal teas. I will strive for good health, happiness and wellness. I will also continue to throw the doona off and stick my feet out, blow up at the smallest thing and wish that I hadn't, feel anxious for no real reason and analyse it for hours. But hopefully these things will become further apart until they slowly disappear.

Ken's story

Ken is Louise's husband. He has generously offered his story as well.

I knew almost nothing about menopause before Lou started. I remember hearing a discussion between my mother and a friend when she was starting to go through it. My only recollection was that it started very early for her—around 42. But no other details. The conversation certainly wasn't with my father.

I had listened to discussions about hormone replacement therapy but I think that was in the context of osteoporosis, and not in any depth about the effects of menopause on women in other physical or mental ways.

Lou and I had never discussed it prior to her starting peri or menopause.

As far as Lou becoming different since menopause, I think change is constant, so I am not sure Lou's personality movement is all to do with her menopause experiences.

Lou and I had choices about our parental roles made for us to a degree. First of all, when our first child was born Lou had a higher income level than me. In a practical sense it would have made sense for me to be the primary caregiver. But from an emotional perspective Lou was the right person to take that role. She wanted it and was best equipped to provide it. We never really discussed Lou going back to work outside the home because not long after Jack was born we moved to Sweden and then the United Kingdom and it was not possible from a visa perspective for Lou to work outside.

I give you this context because I believe menopause comes at a very shitty time for women who have focused on child-rearing and home. It seems to happen when kids are becoming more and more independent and relying less on their parents. So all the physical and mental challenges of menopause for Lou combined with this feeling that her last twenty years of work was becoming less important.

My work has always seen me travel quite a lot and at this time I was establishing myself in a new role. This meant Lou's time alone increased.

Because of this, Lou focused on a relatively new vocation of floristry. This has helped Lou considerably as it gives her a sense of achievement that she needed.

As I said before, I am not sure that all the changes in Lou are about menopause, but in her early fifties she is more controlled emotionally and more likely to cut the world and its inhabitants some slack.

The biggest challenge for me I think at the time was the decrease in sexual activity. Without knowing the effects of menopause on a woman's mind and body my reaction to Lou's decreased desire was to take it personally. Questions like, what about my intimate needs? etc. I know it seems selfish, but for many men their perception of themselves and their sexual activity are intricately linked.

I know now that it wasn't about me, but it felt like it at the time. I hope that my boys will have a better insight into their partners' menopause than I did. I haven't talked it through with them but I will at a later time in their lives.

Most of our conversations about menopause and what Lou was feeling were held at three or four in the morning, when the heat from her body would wake us both up. They were more about the physical effect on her and how it was absolutely doing her head in. Before menopause Lou was very fit; during the menopause I think she was often so tired she didn't have the energy or inclination to exercise. This was then compounding her feelings. Since she has come out the other side, her enthusiasm for exercise has returned and she is even stronger today than before.

On the positive side, Lou is a much more confident person. I think having gone through the changes, she feels like she can achieve anything she sets her mind and body to. What doesn't kill you makes you stronger.

If I was to offer partners any advice it would be to learn about the symptoms and all the possible changes that could occur to your partner. You can't solve this for her, you have to listen and acknowledge. This is not about you at all, even though you will be affected and your relationship will change.

In general men are solvers not listeners. In this case that won't help.

The change in your sexual life will happen and you need to deal with it together.

Looking back, I did learn that I think we could/should have discussed the impacts on us beforehand and/or during. As in any situation in marriage, ignoring a problem will not solve it and it will fester.

I learned a lot about the way Lou was thinking about her life. Her concerns about her position in the world, her achievements and what she wanted to achieve with the rest of it. I hope Lou also learned more about me in this regard.

The best way I found to assist Lou was to listen and encourage.

What I needed from Lou at the time was a better understanding about what the changes in our sexual relationship meant to and for me. Because this thing was happening to Lou sometimes her focus was rightly only on her. It affected us as a couple as well and I think an acknowledgement of that or some warning that it was coming would have helped us.

A delightful postmenopausal zest story

I was one of the fortunate ones whose periods stopped for
eighteen months, then returned only once or twice and then
stopped completely. I was very happy when they stopped
altogether. I wasn't planning on having more children, so I
didn't have to deal with any sense of loss when they ended.
At the height of my suffering, I attended a menopause
support day with other women in my local community. One
woman there who was already in full menopause mentioned
that we would get through it and said that we could look
forward to experiencing a 'post-menopausal zest' when we
got through to the other side. I laughed when she said it and
thought, that doesn't seem very likely. But she was so right—
now I'm there—insomnia gone, full of energy, no more
night sweats, only very occasional flushes and a new-found
confidence and stronger sense of self. I'm enjoying looking
after myself during this stage of life.[5]

Nichole Villeneuve

Celebrities go through menopause

Tell your girlfriends, tell everyone: J.Lo, she's probably in it
now. Sofia Vergara, in it *now*. While I didn't get to sit with these
celebrities, in this article in *Everyday Health* they have shared a
little about their experience with menopause.[6]

Gillian Anderson

When the *X-Files* actress was dealing with the hormonal transition at age 46 in 2017, she wasn't at all sure what was happening to her. 'It was at the point that I felt like my life was falling apart around me that I started to ask what could be going on internally, and friends suggested it might be hormonal,' she recalled in an interview published in March 2017 by *Lenny Letter*, ahead of the release of her book, *We: A Manifesto for Women Everywhere*. 'I was used to being able to balance a lot of things, and all of a sudden I felt like I could handle nothing. I felt completely overwhelmed,' says the actress who portrays a sex therapist in the Netflix series *Sex Education*. 'How wonderful would it be if we could get to a place where we are able to have these conversations openly and without shame,' Anderson says. 'Admit, freely, that this is what's going on. So we don't feel like we're going mad or insane or alone in any of the symptoms we are having.'

Cheryl Hines

Emmy-nominated comedic actress Cheryl Hines has definitely not been curbing her enthusiasm for starting a conversation about painful sex after menopause, often due to vaginal dryness and lack of oestrogen. As the paid spokeswoman for Painfully Awkward Conversations, a campaign sponsored by the makers of medicine for sexual function and menopause-related issues, she urges women to address the issue with their healthcare providers—because there is treatment—and to talk to other women for support.

'It is helpful to talk about it with your friends, so you know other people are dealing with it. The reason a lot of women don't talk to their healthcare providers is because they think they are alone with this,' says Hines.

Angelina Jolie

In March 2015, the actress and activist wrote in *The New York Times* that she had chosen to have her ovaries and fallopian tubes removed because of genetically being at high risk for ovarian cancer. (She also opted for a preventive double mastectomy in 2013 because she carries the BRCA1 gene linked to breast cancer.) The procedure threw her into premature menopause, but Jolie was unwavering about her decision. 'Regardless of the hormone replacements I'm taking, I am now in menopause. I will not be able to have any more children, and I expect some physical changes. But I feel at ease with whatever will come, not because I am strong but because this is a part of life. It is nothing to be feared.'

And when she spoke to the *Daily Telegraph* in an interview in November 2015, she'd had no change of heart. 'I actually love being in menopause,' she said. 'I haven't had a terrible reaction to it, so I'm very fortunate. I feel older, and I feel settled being older. I feel happy that I've grown up. I don't want to be young again.'

Your story

I wish that I could sit down with you and have a cup of tea and ask you questions about you and your symptoms. You've read other women's stories about this time in their lives, and I'd love to know what yours is. Only you can fill in this part; only you know where you've come from, what your life and journey have been as a woman. Looking back at what the women in your family have taught you either consciously or unconsciously, what would you want to tell your younger self about menopause?

How do you want the young women in your life to step into menopause? And now, what do you visualise your life looking like from here on in?

CHAPTER 9

Help

The negative stigma around menopause means that you may go through it without adequate medical or psychological support. Finding the best support and information will assist you to better manage the physical and emotional rollercoaster of menopause.

It goes without saying that you should always seek medical advice before beginning any kind of remedies or medications, or making any drastic lifestyle changes, to ensure the treatments are right for you.

It's reassuring when you find the right doctor for you. A doctor you feel comfortable with, and someone you're confident can connect you to the right treatment for your specific symptoms.

No one knows your body as well as you, and while you may be feeling like a completely different human, trust yourself and know what you feel comfortable taking. Even if you are having symptoms that may seem unrelated, talk about them.

Book an appointment specifically about your symptoms. Allow yourself a good chunk of time to fully disclose everything you are experiencing.

Trust your gut if the medical professional is not the right fit for you. Do you feel this person is listening to you?

There are stories of doctors passing off symptoms of menopause as 'nothing to be concerned about'. Sure, they may not be life-threatening, but some symptoms can cause a huge change in your wellbeing and quality of life.

Questions to consider. Does the physician come recommended? Do you feel cared for in their presence? Don't be afraid to look for a second opinion and find someone better suited to your needs.

Check in with other women and your girlfriends and see if they have any good recommendations for you.

Be ready with a list of your symptoms and the approximate time they started; the more information you give your doctor, the more they can help you. Ask questions! What are the risks, benefits, side effects from any or all of the treatments you might be recommended?

Depending on what type of healer you go to (naturopath, Western medicine, Chinese medicine, etc.), ask if there are other ideas they have—exercise, lifestyle or diet changes—that might also assist you.

I visited my naturopath and my chiropractor/kinesiologist at different times. Both gave me excellent advice and assistance. Both happened to be women, though that does not mean male doctors can't be understanding as well.

There are multiple natural remedies for all sorts of menopausal symptoms. Everything from sleeplessness to mood swings, itchy skin and hot flushes. Even though they are natural, please consult your doctor or naturopath before taking any of the remedies below; we all respond differently to different herbs.

Remember, ladies, you are not your menopause, and your menopause is not you. The physical and mental symptoms you are experiencing will get better with time! This too shall pass . . .

A

Acupuncture

Acupuncture is generally seen as better than no treatment in the management of menopausal symptoms. Individual anecdotal evidence can be quite positive and some evidence suggests that menopausal symptoms such as the incidence and severity of hot flushes may improve with acupuncture.[1] Studies have also shown that acupuncture combined with better nutrition can help manage obesity, which may in turn help with the management of menopausal symptoms.[2]

Adrenal glands

During perimenopause and menopause, the ovaries fluctuate in producing oestrogen and progesterone, which leads to the intermittent nature of the symptoms of menopause.

The adrenal glands produce many different hormones that are pivotal throughout life to the wellbeing of both sexes. For women, the major role that the adrenal hormones play includes physical and mental wellbeing, aging, menstruation and sexual function. If the adrenal glands are not functioning well, hormone levels can drop, negatively impacting a woman's mental and physical health. Studies show that women who show symptoms of exhaustion may be more likely to have a negative experience of perimenopause and menopause. It is important that women take care of their health so that their adrenal glands are functioning well before entering perimenopause.

The hugely popular Dr Axe[3] website includes the following very helpful list of nutrient-dense, low-sugar superfoods that contain healthy fats and fibre for optimal adrenal health:

- coconut
- olives
- avocado and other healthy fats
- cruciferous vegetables (cauliflower, broccoli, Brussels sprouts, etc.)
- fatty fish (e.g., wild-caught salmon)
- free-range chicken and turkey
- bone broth
- nuts, such as walnuts and almonds
- seeds, such as pumpkin, chia and flax
- kelp and seaweed
- Celtic or Himalayan sea salt
- fermented foods rich in probiotics
- chaga and cordyceps medicinal mushrooms.

Affirmations

I love affirmations, I believe in them. I trust they work, I've seen them work, yet I can get so lazy with them. I forget about how powerful they can be. I've stuck Post-it Notes to myself on the mirror to remind myself what words I want to repeat to myself daily. I wanted to include a section in the book about them because of how much I hope they work for you!

I know the attitude with which we embark upon this transition in our lives can have a tremendous impact on our experience of menopause. Countless studies prove negative beliefs held prior to any experience will be more predictive of a difficult time; this is the same for menopause.

On the flipside it has also been shown that changing those negative thoughts and attitudes can result in a reduction of symptoms. Even in the face of difficult symptoms, women consistently say that changing their outlook helps.

This is where affirmations come in. It's a beautiful way to give your mind something else to focus on.

Affirmations plus actions equals miracles.

Esther Hicks
....

What I understand is, when you feel uncomfortable and negative it's better to seek out happier feelings like this one:

My body is vital and healthy.

I do believe there is a power inside our bodies that has the ability to change and heal. One way to heal is in the way we think.

When I was growing up, one of the worst accusations was that you 'loved yourself', it was hurled at you if you spoke too highly of something you had achieved, looked in the mirror for too long, or didn't crumble under an assault against how you looked.

But loving yourself has nothing to do with vanity. It's the total opposite. I'm learning the fastest journey to loving myself is to look for appreciation in everything I see, including me.

I heard this affirmation and loved it.

I love myself therefore I take loving care of my body.

Louise Hay
. . . .

The universe loves grateful people. The more grateful you are the more you get to be grateful about.

Louise Hay
. . . .

Some other affirmations that I have on hand are:

I love myself just the way I am.
All my relationships are harmonious.
I listen with love to my body's messages.
I express gratitude for all that I have in my life.
My body now restores to its natural state of good health.

Changing your outlook from the negative to the positive creates a whole different reality.

You have the ability to change your life with a change of perception.

Sometimes the first step in changing my perception is just saying I CAN instead of I CAN'T.

It's like planting a seed in the ground. It might not be something I necessarily believe right now, but I have a goal to eventually believe and live it.

Tell your close friends your affirmation and goals so they can support you. That way they know what your intention is. Beware the people who want to ridicule or quash your desire. Don't even mention it to them—it's like going to the mechanic to get your nails done.

Anthroposophic medicine

Anthroposophic medicine is an integrative multimodal treatment system based on a holistic understanding of humans and nature and of disease and treatment.[4] It builds on a concept of four levels of formative forces and on the model of a three-fold human constitution.

There is a related, larger shift that many women experience at menopause, when a new experience or awareness of self emerges—often on a social (community), artistic or spiritual level—because the forces that have previously, repeatedly, been given outside of oneself are now available inwardly. Then the 'bounty' of forces needs a new direction. A new balance is found between inside and outside, between physically mothering (premenopausal) and spiritually nurturing (postmenopausal). It is a doorway out of physiologic devotion, but with the possibility of new wisdom.

Ayurvedic

Ayurveda is a system of traditional medicine that teaches that prevention is always the best course of action, so getting things in shape premenopause is, of course, preferable.

Kester Marshall, Ayurvedic practitioner and naturopath says, 'Simple herbal remedies can help enormously to smooth the balance of hormones and reduce flushes during this transition; and in more extreme situations where a lot of toxins and deeper imbalances have surfaced, stronger cleansing programs can be of great benefit.'

Ayurvedic treatments will also help in both the lead-up to menopause and in reducing difficult menopausal symptoms.

Menopause is a perfectly natural and very gradual process with oestrogen levels often taking many years to decrease.[5]

B

Balance

My dear friend, who is a nutritionist, says she recommends everything in moderation. Meaning, you don't have to cut out every single scrap of sugar from your diet. Having a glass of wine every now and then is okay. As long as you are eating well and balanced you can still enjoy the yummy things in life!

Basil oil

There are so many wonderful essential oils that assist in menopause. One of them, basil oil, is an energising oil that you can use topically or in aromatherapy to improve your focus and fatigue.

Belief system

What's your belief about menopause? Are you avoiding it by not talking about it? Are you embarrassed about being in menopause? Do you believe you have been possessed by a vindictive demon that is robbing you of everything you love? Are you embracing the changes and know that this is a wonderful time for you to be 100 per cent you?

> Apologise to your body. Maybe that's where the healing begins.
>
> *Nayyirah Waheed*

Black cohosh

Black cohosh has been used for centuries by Native Americans in the treatment of menstrual irregularities, menopause symptoms, and to ease childbirth. Always talk to your doctor before taking black cohosh as it has been linked to liver failure in some studies.

Reduces hot flush

Over the years, research has cast doubt upon the efficacy of black cohosh for managing symptoms of menopause. More recently, however, data has been more promising when studies have looked at the impact of black cohosh and hot flushes.[6] Taking it regularly reduces the number and severity of hot flushes, bringing huge relief to the high percentage of menopausal women who report experiencing these symptoms.

Aids sleep

Sleep is vital to balancing hormones naturally throughout life, as a lack of sleep disturbs hormone production and management. Many women report sleep disturbance as a symptom of menopause. Sleep is particularly important as the effects of other menopause symptoms are compounded through sleep disturbance.

A small study in 2015 looked at the role of black cohosh in postmenopausal women with sleep problems and had promising results.[7] Further trials in this would need to be conducted to understand whether black cohosh can alleviate sleep problems in postmenopausal women.

Sleeping at the right time is just as vital to women experiencing sleeplessness during menopause as the length of time (seven to eight hours) that is recommended. The right time, according to endocrinologists (hormone experts), includes the four hours between 10 p.m. and 2 a.m. This will ensure the most effective and hormonally balanced sleep.

Breasts

Here are eight natural ways to manage breast tenderness in menopause that work.

Breast tenderness in menopause can be quite uncomfortable, but the good news is that it's highly manageable.

1. Give your boobs some loving attention

When one or both of your 'girls' feel tender, one way to calm them down is through breast massage. Breast massaging has many benefits, including:

- improves blood circulation
- reduces swelling
- promotes lymphatic drainage and flushing out of toxins
- releases tension and tightness
- maintains the shape of the breasts and increases their size
- helps in pain relief, easing soreness
- increases your sensitivity, intensifying pleasure and improving orgasm
- stimulates the release of youthful hormones
- triggers the production of oxytocin (love hormone), reducing stress and depression.

2. Use oils

To add more positive effects to breast massage, use oils with essential fatty acids to help decrease breast pain. Olive oil and coconut oil are rich in gamma-linolenic acid (an essential fatty acid), which has anti-inflammatory and analgesic effects. Just take a few drops of this oil and apply it gently on your breasts for pain relief.

3. *Fill your body with vitamins and minerals*

Vitamins B, C and E have anti-inflammatory and antioxidant properties. They also have balancing effects, which can help your hormones in correcting premenstrual syndrome (PMS). Here are some foods rich in these vitamins:

- vitamin B—salmon, chicken breast, avocado, spinach and hazelnuts
- vitamin C—citrus fruits like orange, lemon and cruciferous veggies
- vitamin E—sweet potato, sunflower seeds, olive oil and butternut pumpkin.

Calcium, magnesium and selenium may also help. Calcium and selenium relax the muscles and maintain nerve health. Foods high in these minerals include:

- magnesium—Swiss chard, figs, pumpkin seeds and dark chocolate
- calcium—chia seeds, leafy greens, hemp milk, almond milk, sesame seeds, fennel, artichoke, broccoli
- selenium—Brazil nuts, shiitake mushrooms, lima beans, sunflower, flax and sesame seeds, cabbage, spinach.

4. Start a hormone-supporting diet

- **Eat high-fibre foods.** Berries, vegetables, legumes and whole grains.
- **Decrease caffeine consumption.** Coffee is good and I'm not saying to totally get rid of it. How about going decaf or replacing your warm coffee with lemon honey water? A compound called methylxanthines are present in coffee, which may contribute to inflammation.
- **Avoid smoking and alcohol consumption.** Cigarette smoke breaks down elastin, a type of protein that maintains firmness of the skin and tissues. For this reason, it is common for the breasts to feel sore when women smoke or consume alcohol.

5. Wear supportive bras

Wear well-fitted and supportive bras instead of underwire bras. To choose the right bra, make sure it cups your breasts well. If you feel tender breasts at night, you may want to wear a bra to bed if it feels comfortable for you. Get rid of old and stretched-out bras because they no longer provide enough support.

6. Move more and maintain your weight

7. Warm and cold packs for immediate relief

For quick relief from breast soreness, you can use moist warm packs on your breasts for a few minutes. You can also take a hot shower to ease the pain. A friendly reminder: don't use your warm packs for more than five minutes because it can increase the swelling. Warm packs will open your blood vessels and improve blood circulation to the breast area. After using warm packs, use a cold compress for about ten minutes to constrict your blood vessels

8. Free your breasts!

Free your breasts from time to time. Although bras can be quite helpful, they can also impede your lymph from flowing freely, which is why you need to give your breasts time to breathe!

When you sleep at night, you can go braless but still support your boobs with a soft pillow. You can also elevate your head a little. This increases blood flow and reduces swelling.

When should I go to the doctor for breast tenderness?

When women hear about breast tenderness in menopause, they immediately think of breast cancer. But the good news is, breast soreness is rarely a symptom of breast cancer. With that said, here are some warning signs that you need to go to your doctor:

- severe and frequent pain with fluid discharge
- breast pain that doesn't go away and which isn't connected to your period
- unusual symptoms, like lumps, nipple discharge, severe swelling and redness
- orange-peel skin
- dimples in the surrounding area of your breast
- numbness in hands or fingers
- chest pain.

I know many women are afraid of breast cancer, but you can take part in your own assessment. A good way to do this is to practise the self-breast exam which you can learn on your own.[8]

C

Citrus oil

So apparently citrus oil has been known to assist with boosting our sexual drive and libido, and as well as its anti-inflammatory properties it can help relieve achy joints make this a winner to have in the bathroom cabinet.[9]

Clary sage oil

Clary sage oil has been known to help with anxiety and depression. It's even believed to have stronger benefits than lavender, as it has some effects on our feel-good hormone, dopamine.[10]

Creativity

Time to get your creative pants on, ladies—they can be sweatpants, by the way, or you can even get creative in your underwear if it's too hot for pants. Just get them on and take that weaving/painting/pottery/writing/rocket-making class.

Crying does not indicate that you are weak. Since birth, it
has always been a sign that you are alive.

Charlotte Bronte

D

Vitamin D

As you know, mood swings can be a common symptom in the menopause years. Vitamin D has been shown to have a positive effect on low mood and cognitive performance. Taking care of our health as we get older is important; vitamin D helps to absorb calcium and build bones to keep us strong. It's also involved in many other processes that protect you from disease and health problems.[11]

> We are dismissed as emotional. It is enough to make you emotional.
>
> *Sara Ahmed,* Living a Feminist Life

E

Evening primrose oil

Evening primrose oil is one of the most popular remedies for menopausal changes. While the evidence is anecdotal, evening primrose oil is said to help with the following menopause-related changes:

- anxiety
- hair loss
- hot flushes
- insomnia

- joint pain
- mood swings
- night sweats
- weight gain.[12]

Extra care

We need to take extra care of ourselves during the shift happening to our bodies: longer baths, quieter mornings, healthier food, longer and more frequent walks. Give yourself the time to care fully and wholeheartedly for yourself.

> Dieting is easy. It's like riding a bike. Except the bike is on fire. And the ground is on fire. And everything is on fire. Because you are in hell.
>
> *Jillian Michael*
> ....

F

Fitness

If you have not already begun to move your body in some way shape or form, it's time. Beginning perimenopause it's a *must*, and it's also a win–win situation. You become healthier all around, plus your symptoms will be way easier to handle. Start small if you need—I started with a simple yoga stretch class and built up till my body could handle the actual yoga poses. I then found other ways to be active: walking group, riding my bike. I've also added dance classes with a friend because: a. it's a great way to get fit and, b. it's absolutely hilarious—if the workout doesn't help, the laughing at least tones the abs and gives me the endorphins I need!

Food

Good foods to eat during menopause

- Apricots, avocados, bananas, sweet potatoes. Why? They're good sources of potassium, which helps regulate blood pressure.
- Berries. Why? They're high in fibre, low in calories and packed with disease-fighting antioxidants.
- Dark, leafy greens. Why? Where to begin . . . how about they're high in fibre and rich in calcium and vitamin K, both of which help support strong bones.
- Iron-rich foods. Why? Hormonal changes conspire against your energy levels, and iron-rich foods are one antidote. A few choices: lean red meats, poultry, fish, kale, spinach, lentils, beans.
- Salmon and other oily fish. Why? They're one of the few good food sources of vitamin D, which your body needs to absorb calcium. Plus, they're high in omega-3 fatty acids, which have been shown to raise good cholesterol.
- Whole grains. Why? In a word: Fibre. Studies show that the soluble fibre in whole grains helps your body remove cholesterol. Plus, it's key to a healthy digestive system. Good choices: oatmeal, whole wheat bread, popcorn, quinoa.

- Yoghurt. Why? It's another good source of calcium, plus it's a good protein choice and contains probiotics for a healthier GI tract. Look for low-sugar varieties, or buy plain yoghurt and add your own sweet or savoury stir-ins.
- Water. Why? Okay, it's not food, but it is necessary to keep your body systems functioning and, hello, it comes in handy during a hot flush.

Friends

Call them, lean on them, share with them. Spend time with people who are good for your mental health.

G

Geranium

Geranium is yet another wonderful oil. Used in a diffuser or applied on the skin mixed with almond oil, it's said to help with night sweats and hydrating the skin.

Good times

Make them, create them, plan for them, take them! Keeping up the good times as you are being challenged in all sorts of ways is so important for your mental health. Make a concerted effort to create fun in your life.

H

Hair

Here are ten nutrients for healthy hair during menopause.

1. Protein

Keratin is a protein and is the building block of your hair, and while it is not directly found in food, its production is directly affected by how much protein is in your diet. A lack of protein in your diet can have a lasting impact on your hair health, especially during perimenopause and menopause. Keratin is made up of amino acids, which your body gets from protein-rich foods such as red meat, beans, fish, eggs and milk, as well as vegetables such as kale and asparagus.

2. Vitamin C

Vitamin C is the nutrient that just keeps on giving and is essential for maintaining healthy hair during menopause. Vitamin C is the common name for ascorbic acid, specifically L-ascorbic acid, and is a small molecule organic acid. This means that when it is added to hair products like shampoo, it can be effective to remove mineral build up and therefore improve your hair's ability to absorb moisture, thereby improving hair health. It is also effective to prevent hair damage as it acts as an antioxidant, which removes free radicals, protecting against structural damage to the proteins in hair.

3. Vitamin A

Another wonder vitamin, Vitamin A, can increase the speed of cell regeneration and synthesis. Therefore, a deficiency can have a direct effect on the maintenance of healthy hair during menopause. It is key for moisturising your hair and preventing it from getting brittle.

4. Fats

There has been debate about how much fat to include in your diet for many years, however it is generally agreed that you need healthy fats in your diet. If you don't, you risk damaging your hair, as these healthy fats provide your body with linoleic acids, along with long-chain polyunsaturated fats, which are essential for hair structure. If you're looking for good fats to include in your diet, fish can be an excellent source, as can flaxseeds and olive oil.

5. Niacin

Niacin is the little-known solution to hair woes and can be an excellent addition when promoting healthy hair during menopause. Niacin is also known as vitamin B_3 or nicotinic acid, and it is a water-soluble vitamin that helps the body convert food into energy and helps maintain the structure of blood cells and improve circulation. It has an effect on hair growth as it can improve blood circulation to the scalp, which in turn brings oxygen and other nutrients to your hair follicles.

6. Pantothenic acid

Pantothenic acid is also known as vitamin B_5 and is very important for healthy hair during menopause. By strengthening the cells in your hair follicles it helps them to work properly and thereby promotes hair growth. Not only that, increasing the amount of vitamin B_5 in your diet can help with issues like dandruff or itchy skin. Good sources of pantothenic acid include egg yolk, fish, beef, brewer's yeast, liver, pork, sweet potatoes and tomatoes.

7. Iron

An iron deficiency can often be the cause of hair loss and therefore during menopause it is essential to consume enough iron in your diet. This will help to ensure healthy hair as, much like niacin, it contributes to increased blood flow to the scalp and therefore improved maintenance of your hair follicles.

8. Vitamin B_{12}

Vitamin B_{12} is another nutrient that helps promote healthy blood flow as it aids in the production of red blood cells. Red blood cells are responsible for carrying oxygen to your tissues, including your hair follicles, and also play a role in maintaining your hair colour. Foods which contain high levels of vitamin B_{12} include meats, fish, eggs and dairy products, which is why women who eat a vegetarian or vegan diet should consider taking a vitamin B_{12} supplement to ensure they don't become deficient.

9. Folate

Folate is another B vitamin that plays an important role in maintaining healthy hair during menopause. It occurs naturally in certain foods, including green peas, white beans, eggs, cod and liver, and can also be found in many supplements. Folate plays a critical role in the growth of hair tissue as it stimulates the rebuilding of your follicle cells. Not only that, it improves blood flow, which as we have already discovered plays a crucial role in hair health.

10. Zinc

Many experts believe that zinc deficiency can lead to the breakdown of the protein structures in your hair follicle, which can lead to hair loss. It is also believed to play an important role in DNA production and can help regulate your hormones, which can be important if your hair loss is indeed caused by a hormonal imbalance. Zinc supplements can be a great way to ensure you get plenty of this particular nutrient, however foods such as oysters, nuts, eggs, chickpeas, sweet potato and spinach are also packed full of it and can be great for maintaining healthy hair during menopause.[13]

Heart palpitations

Heart palpitations, also known as rapid heartbeat or heart flutter, are another common occurrence at menopause due to changing hormones. They can feel scary, and shouldn't be overlooked if you feel you need some extra advice from your doctor to make sure what you are experiencing is just hormonal changes and not something else. In an article, Dr Northrup suggests that our 'midlife hearts' become very sensitive and are alerting us to what no longer serve us: drugs, alcohol, and eating crap foods that may overstimulate our hearts.[14]

Homeopathy

There are no specific medicines for oestrogen dominance, low progesterone or hormone replacement therapy (HRT) in homeopathy.

Homeopathy works in a different way, addressing issues holistically. Hormone imbalance also causes many changes in the emotional plane. Hormones can change our mood and behaviour. Additional stress may also occur due to weight gain, skin problems like acne, or facial hair.

Homeopathy treats the person having a hormonal imbalance. Homeopathy addresses both emotional and physical issues. There are many remedies in homeopathy that match the symptom picture of persons with hormonal imbalance.

A homeopathic pharmacy can offer a wide range of medicines that could be appropriate for patients with menopausal reactions.[15]

Hormone replacement therapy (HRT)

What is hormone replacement therapy?

As the name implies, hormone replacement therapy (HRT) is a replacement of female sex hormones in women. These hormones are called oestrogen and progesterone. They are released from the ovaries and influence changes in the body's cycle that controls periods, moods and may contribute to a sense of wellbeing and healthiness. Oestrogen is also very important to maintain strong, healthy bones. Usually every month in a healthy woman of childbearing age hormones are produced and released from the brain and pituitary gland to encourage one of her two ovaries to produce an egg (ovum). At the same time oestrogen and progesterone are released from the ovaries, which cause changes that help to prepare the body for pregnancy.

If pregnancy does not occur the hormone levels fall and the woman will have a period. After menopause the ovaries no longer respond to the hormones from the pituitary gland and shut down. This means a woman can no longer become pregnant naturally and her periods stop. This is when symptoms may appear, including hot flushes, night sweats, insomnia, palpitations, mood changes, vaginal dryness and painful intercourse, and mild skin changes, such as dryness and loss of elasticity. Treating patients with HRT replaces the hormones no longer being released from the ovary and some of these symptoms can be helped.

When can hormone replacement therapy be used?

Most women have their menopause between 50 and 55 years of age. Some women go into an early menopause before they are 45. In these women HRT can be used before the age of 50 without increasing their risk of breast cancer. Most women are postmenopausal by 54. The symptoms of menopause may last any time from one to five years, and some women still experience hot flushes some ten years after their menopause began. Some may not have hot flushes at all.

What types of therapy are there?

HRT can be given by tablets, patches, creams or gels under advice from a GP. HRT can take different forms:

- oestrogen only; for women who do not have a uterus (womb)
- cyclical combined—which is oestrogen and progesterone together and reintroduces monthly periods
- continuous combined—these prevent periods and may either be oestrogen and progesterone combined or Tibolone—a synthetic medication that has combined effects of oestrogen, progesterone and testosterone.

Women with an intact uterus must take combined HRT, replacing both oestrogen and progesterone, to prevent the lining of the womb thickening and thus reducing the risk of endometrial cancer of the womb.

If a woman has had a hysterectomy then therapy can be oestrogen only. If she has already been on a cyclical combined course of therapy and reaches 54 years of age, or has had no periods for 12 months before starting HRT, she should start continuous combined HRT to prevent regular monthly bleeds.

The current recommended form of HRT is body-identical HRT, which usually involves an oestrogen gel and a capsule of micronised progesterone inserted into the uterus (if the woman has one). If you are on a cyclical regime, it will be two capsules a day for twelve days of your cycle and a continuous regime is one capsule per day throughout the month. This is the safest and most commonly prescribed regime as it is cardiovascularly protective, though should not be started for cardiovascular protection alone.

For how long can hormone replacement therapy be given and what are the risks?

The current recommendations are for the lowest dose for the shortest possible time to control symptoms. Women who do not have symptoms of menopause should not use HRT. All types of HRT are linked with a small increase in the risk of breast cancer and some therapies increase the risk of cancer of the uterus. After five years of continuous HRT there is an increased risk of ovarian cancer, with research indicating one extra case of ovarian cancer for every 8000 women taking HRT each year. The risk of breast cancer depends on age but increases with the length of the therapy.

As an example, a woman aged 50 has a 6.1 per cent risk of getting breast cancer in the next 30 years. If she takes oestrogen-only HRT for five years, the risk is 6.28 per cent. If she takes combined HRT (oestrogen and progesterone) for three years, the risk rises to 6.4 per cent. If she takes it for five years, it increases to 6.7 per cent, and for ten years to 7.69 per cent.

There are some benefits of HRT, including strengthening the bones, which reduces the risk of osteoporosis and broken bones, but this is only during the time of taking HRT. HRT also reduces the risk of getting bowel cancer but does not prevent heart disease, strokes or dementia. HRT should not be used for long-term protection of osteoporosis.

Women newly started on HRT should have their symptoms reviewed by their doctor after three months. Women who then remain on HRT should be reviewed at least every year by their doctor to see whether continuing on HRT is still the best treatment for them.[16]

Hot flushes and ways to cool them

Add aromatherapy

Clary sage and Roman chamomile essential oils help balance mood swings, while peppermint can chill hot flush. To make your own cooling mist (especially great for night sweats!), mix the following ingredients in a 120 millilitre dark-glass spray bottle:

90 ml distilled water

30 ml witch hazel extract

8 drops each of peppermint, clary sage, and Roman chamomile essential oils

Breathe deep and slow

Take full, deep, slow breaths. Research has found that when we stress, the hot flushes are worse. Makes sense, right? So whether you meditate or just listen to calming music, reducing your stress will help the hot flush.

Sip some sage

Because sage may have oestrogen-like effects, avoid therapeutic amounts if you've had breast cancer or could be pregnant. I've found sage tea at my local health food store. It's actually a really pleasant-tasting tea. You can brew it and leave it to get cold, adding ice cubes to give it that cooling effect when having a hot flush. Have two to three cups a day.

I

Iron

Iron deficiencies are common in premenopausal women who get their menstrual periods each month. This is because iron is lost through the blood on regular cycles. Since postmenopausal women eventually no longer get their periods, many do not lose as much iron as they did before over time. However, postmenopausal women who are iron deficient need to be investigated by their doctor to exclude bowel cancer.

Iron needs after menopause

Once a woman reaches menopause, a lack of iron can lead to many other conditions that are uncomfortable, embarrassing, and even degenerative. Some studies have linked iron to hot flushes, and people with iron deficiencies often report poor cold intolerance and body temperature regulation.

Osteoporosis is another major concern among women of menopausal age, and an iron deficiency can affect bone density. This is essential to keeping bones healthy and strong throughout the aging process. Women going through menopause often experience fatigue, and this could be due to an iron deficiency as well.[17]

I'm still inventing myself, so it's not over till it's over.

Hadley Boyd[18]
....

Itching during menopause

During menopause, oestrogen production decreases, and this decrease can cause itching. Oestrogen stimulates the production of natural oils and collagen—a protein responsible for skin strength and elasticity—which help keep skin moist. So during menopause, skin is susceptible to becoming drier and thinner, which can make it feel itchy.

You may have found you have a sensitivity to certain soaps and moisturisers that you didn't use to have a problem with, or that your skin is thinner, flaky or red. Of course, see a doctor if your skin is irritated so that you can rule out other forms of skin irritation, such as bacterial or fungal infections.

Genital itching

Low levels of oestrogen can also affect the vaginal tissues by making them drier and thinner than before. The following factors can also cause vaginal itching:

- irritation from soaps or detergents
- inflammation
- vaginal, vulvar, or rarely, cervical cancers.

Make sure you see your doctor if you notice any vaginal discharge or vaginal bleeding after menopause to rule out certain cancers.

Home remedies

There are some things you can do to ease the discomfort of itchy skin:

- Apply liberal amounts of moisturiser regularly, and at least twice a day. Moisturising can relieve dryness and itching. Personally, I've never moisturised as much as I have in the last few years. I do this as soon as I wake up and of course when I go to bed and often times in between. My skin laps it up. The best time to apply moisturiser is after a bath or shower, when the skin is still slightly damp, as this can help to lock moisture into the outermost layer of the skin. Almond oil, jojoba oil and shea butter are all great, natural choices.
- Apply a cool, wet compress to areas where you skin is irritated.
- Take an oatmeal bath. If you have kids you probably have already bathed your little ones in oatmeal—it's a great skin soother. Simply cut the leg off some old pantyhose and put rolled oats into it, tie the end off in a knot and immerse it into your bath water. Or get hold of colloidal oatmeal, which is oatmeal in a fine powder form and add this to your bath water. Avoid using hot water, as hot baths can make the itchiness worse.

- Use a humidifier if you live in an area that has a dry climate. Or if you work in an air-conditioned building, as air-conditioning removes moisture from the air.
- Use skin-friendly laundry detergents that don't contain any added colour or fragrance.
- Supplement with fish oil, which has been shown to improve skin hydration. Think of it as moisturising from within.

Preventing itchiness during menopause

You can reduce the likelihood of itchy skin during menopause by doing the following:

- Stay hydrated by drinking adequate amounts of water throughout the day. It's one of the easiest ways to keep skin moist and supple.
- Swap hot baths and showers for lukewarm ones instead. Hot water can strip the skin of its natural oils.
- Keep your showers and baths short to avoid drying out your skin.
- Pat yourself dry with a soft towel after a bath or shower— don't rub. Rubbing skin dry after a bath or shower can irritate already sore, sensitive or itchy skin.
- Try not to scratch your itchy skin—you risk injuring it further. If you suspect you're scratching your skin in your sleep, wearing light cotton gloves to bed can help.
- Check the label of your skincare products. Perfumes are a common ingredient in cleansers and moisturisers, and they can irritate skin. Even products marketed as natural can contain

irritating ingredients. Looking for products labelled as suitable for sensitive skin is a safer option.

- Reduce your intake of alcohol and nicotine. Alcohol in particular can be very dehydrating and both alcohol and nicotine can age the skin prematurely.
- Choose cotton and natural fibres. Cotton is much less irritating to the skin than either wool or synthetic fibres; plus cotton and natural fibres breathe better than synthetics.
- Wear soft, loose-fitting clothes as they are less likely to irritate skin than close-fitting clothes.
- Be UV aware. The harmful UV rays in sunlight can irritate dry, itchy, or sensitive skin. Using a high-SPF sunblock suitable for sensitive skin is best for your skin.[19]

What I've been doing

Add Glow from SWIISH to your nightly cup of sleep and you've got yourself a cocktail of goodness. Glow helps with rebuilding collagen, which starts to decline as we get older. This completely solved my itchy face along with Thalia Skin's The Awakening Serum—a gorgeous mix of organic oils that calmed my skin. I also often add a slather of Jojoba oil and Egyptian Magic cream to keep my skin feeling moisturised. The changes in my body . . . it's a journey of self-love. I wear my clothes looser; I want to feel good, comfortable, stylish, but most of all *comfortable*.

J

Joint pain

Menopause and perimenopause can result in joint pain. Other factors such as wear and tear, obesity, stress, loss of muscle, inactivity, injury and certain diseases contribute to joint pain. Dehydration and an increase in the levels of uric acid may cause inflammation.

Remedies for joint pain include a healthy diet. Fresh fruit and vegetables, wholegrains, nuts and dried fruit that contain magnesium are beneficial. Calcium, which can be taken as a supplement, is helpful and is aided in absorption by a sufficient intake of magnesium. You can take supplements of magnesium and calcium. Low-impact exercise, such as swimming, Pilates or yoga, can help. Avoiding high-impact exercise, such as jogging on hard surfaces, can make a difference in reducing the incidence of joint pain.[20]

Joking

That's right, humour and self-deprecation and not taking ourselves too seriously are all super-useful strategies too many of us often overlook . . . probably because we're taking life too seriously.

How does this help? There are numerous explanations but one of the more compelling is that humour essentially helps us see things from a different perspective, more often than not a lighter, less serious and hopefully more helpful perspective. Notably, something very similar is at the heart of many contemporary psychological therapies, including cognitive-behavioural approaches and acceptance and commitment therapies.

So find a way to laugh at yourself, especially at your stressors and troubles. Seeing some things as silly might secure a path towards resilience and even happiness.[21]

K

Kindness

Never underestimate the impact of kindness and its power to heal. Kindness to yourself at this time is imperative. Your body is not your enemy.

L

Lavender oil

Oh boy, do I love lavender. Not only for its scent but how it can assist with insomnia and helping me to relax and get the rest I need. Lavender is well studied for its capabilities and is safer than sleeping pills and medication for sleeplessness.[22]

Love

Love yourself through this time. If you don't, why should anyone else? Love the new chapter, the new you. Love the feeling of freedom and the blossoming of a wiser, more wonderful you.

M

Magnesium

Eight ways magnesium rescues hormones, according to Lara Briden, the author of *Hormone Repair Manual*:

1. Regulates cortisol. It calms your nervous system and prevents excessive cortisol. Your stress hormonal system—also called your hypothalamic-pituitary-adrenal (HPA) axis— is your central hormonal system. When it functions well, then your other hormones (thyroid and reproductive hormones) will function well too.

2. Reduces blood sugar and normalises insulin. It's so effective at improving insulin sensitivity that Briden refers to magnesium as 'natural metformin'. Healthy insulin sensitivity means fewer sugar cravings and is effective treatment for weight loss and PCOS.

3. Supports thyroid. Magnesium is essential for the production of thyroid hormone. It is also anti-inflammatory, which helps to quiet the autoimmune inflammation that underlies most thyroid disease. Other ways to address thyroid autoimmunity include gluten-elimination and a selenium supplement.

4. Aids sleep. Magnesium is the great sleep-promoter, and sleep is crucial for hormone production. Sleep is when we should enjoy a beneficial surge of anabolic hormones such as DHEA and growth hormone.

5. Fuels cellular energy. It's so intricately involved with mitochondria and energy production, that we can safely say, without

magnesium, there is no cellular energy. Hormonal tissue has a high metabolic rate, and so requires even more cellular energy and more magnesium than other tissue.

6. Makes hormones. It aids in the manufacture of steroid hormones, including progesterone, oestrogen, and testosterone. That may be why magnesium has been shown to reduce hot flushes by 50 per cent.
7. Activates vitamin D. Without enough magnesium, vitamin D cannot do its job. Conversely, too much vitamin D supplementation causes magnesium deficiency.
8. Slows aging. It prevents telomere shortening, reduces oxidative stress, and enhances the production of glutathione.[23]

Masturbation

I've read this over and over from sex therapists to women struggling with intimacy with their significant other.

Masturbate.

Explore what feels good to you. If you have pain every time you have sex, why would you do it? Buy the lube, or use coconut oil. I've heard it said, 'If you don't use it, you lose it.' The actual orgasm is good for the vagina, it's like a little fitness class, activating blood cells in the vagina. The walls of the vagina thin as we age. Keeping the vagina healthy and happy is key to our sexual health. It can also help to kickstart your libido again.

Meditation

In an insightful article written by Ellen Dolgen, she observes the power and benefits of meditation. You've seen the pictures before:

A woman sitting cross-legged, her hands gently resting on her knees. She looks so peaceful. Ooooom.

You can attain this with a few simple steps!

According to the American Psychological Association, simply changing one's focus to more meditative mindfulness can help improve our mental clarity, emotional intelligence and our ability to relate to others with kindness, acceptance and compassion. Sign me up!

During stressful times it can feel like we are always in fight or flight mode. Kinda feels like we are being chased by a lion all day. This can play havoc on our health and add to menopausal stress, which can contribute to memory loss, weight gain and overall aging.

According to the American Heart Association, stress may contribute to poor health behaviours linked to an increased risk for heart disease and stroke, such as overeating, lack of physical activity, back strain, stomach pains, zapped energy and lack of sleep, and it can make you feel cranky and out of control. Sound familiar?! Luckily, calming your heart can seriously quiet all that stress buzzing through your mind. Here is where mindfulness and meditation enter the picture!

When we relax, our heart rate slows down. But when we meditate, the interval between each beat of our heart changes and becomes smoother. That interval between each beat is called Heart Rate Variability (or HRV), and smoothing it out is what lets those yogi masters live longer—in fact, in 2010, the *American Journal of Cardiology* reported that maintaining a healthy HRV as we age actually predicts longevity!

So now that you are motivated to meditate, here are three quick and easy meditations from Andy Puddicombe, founder of *headspace.com*, for finding menopausal bliss.

1. On the road

Flip road rage the bird! Sit up straight and focus on your butt pressing against the seat. Start by listening to the sounds around you—the wheels on the road, the purr of the motor—then focus on each of your other senses for a minute. Next, tune into them all, letting them come together in your mind like the parts of an orchestra. And here's the key: Instead of seeing yourself as being affected (aka stressed) by it, think about how you are a part of this ever-changing environment.

2. During lunch

Do you eat your lunch—or inhale it? If you're busy (and who isn't?), lunch can become just another thing you multitask. Instead, consider being a bit more mindful of your meal. Before digging in, spend a couple of minutes doing nothing, just relaxing and leaving the day's stress behind. Then, make like an *Iron Chef* judge and pay attention to what you're eating. How does the food taste and feel in your mouth? How does it make you feel?

3. In bed

Lie in bed with your eyes closed (easy!). Now, rather than pass out (or toss and turn if that's more your style), breathe deeply. Starting at your toes—and working all the way to the tip of your noggin, focus on each body part. Relax each muscle like you're powering down your phone before a flight. (This really works—I've been doing it for years. You can do this at your desk, too!)

You don't need to have candles and incense lit to meditate. You can take a no-frills approach to meditation; it can become part of many happier, healthier, and stress-free days to come.[24]

Mood swings

What can you do for yourself at home when you feel those mood swings take hold? I'm going to sound like a broken record, though it's been proven to help: EXERCISE.

Find a way to release those endorphins. Blast your favourite song as you vacuum the house and dance at the same time. You don't need to be training like an Olympic athlete, find the time of day that suits you best and stick to a four-day-a-week plan of moving your body. Studies have shown that hot flushes, irritability and mood swings have all been lessened when we release the feel-good endorphins in our brain. So get moving any way you can!

Letting go of stress . . . easier said than done, right? Stress is something I have to consciously tackle—it won't disappear on its own. It might go into hiding for a while, but it begins to show up in my body and my moods. Again, finding ways to help you release your stress is imperative, whether it's a walk in nature, a swim in the ocean, meditation, yoga, a good book, scrabble with your kids, or watching a comedy. Whatever helps, Do. It. More.

As mentioned previously, the big key to mood swings is sleep. Check out the tips later in this chapter and try some of them. Fingers crossed for a good seven to eight hours' sleep.

When to seek help

I have taken myself off to see a therapist for my mood swings; please go visit someone you trust if you are feeling any of the below symptoms:

- extreme mood swings
- extra anxiety
- moods that are making it difficult to participate fully in life.

Maybe keep a diary of your mood swings, including any possible triggers. What activities you've been up to, whether there were stressful situations, what foods you are eating and if you are taking any medications or supplements.

What I've been using

I've seen a therapist for many years now. When my marriage was falling apart I gratefully found an incredible person to assist me with the pain I was feeling. So when I felt the gaping hole of depression beckoning me forth I knew I needed support again. I also really needed to talk with someone that wasn't my husband, I needed another set of ears to pour out all of my crazy, sad, depressed, angry feelings. Hearing them out loud was so helpful, rather than having them rattling around like a trapped bird in my head.

I have always found writing in a journal incredibly helpful. It does not have to be done religiously, just when the emotions feel so overwhelming that you feel you can't move on. Giving myself a break, some quiet time, helps me deal with my emotions, as does taking a walk with a friend. And laughter is, as they say, the best medicine—all those magical endorphins that get released when we laugh are one of the best ways to beat the blues.

One of the best soothing remedies for me has been my dogs. Spending time with animals opens my heart like nothing else. My dogs don't care about the new hairs sprouting from my chin, or my hot flushes. They love me when I'm sad or happy. In fact, on days when I've cried my dogs seek me out and just sit next to me like a good friend. Never do I feel judged, just loved. So if you feel yourself spinning out of control, maybe go pat an animal and see if that helps.

I believe the second half of one's life is meant to be better than the first half. The first half is finding out how you do it. And the second half is enjoying it.

Frances Lear
....

N

Nature

Go into nature; there is magic waiting for you in the natural world, all you need to do is go out into it. Nature can quickly shift the way I'm feeling—swimming in the ocean, or even sitting on the beach, or taking a walk in a green environment and breathing the air that trees create is a magical solution for a stressed mind and body.

In an interview on mine and Cam's podcast, 'Separate Bathrooms', Indigenous man Mitch Tambo spoke so beautifully about how 'being on country' can help with our mental health. Even for those of us who are not of Indigenous lineage, respectfully heading into nature and lying on green grass or putting our bare feet in the earth or, as Mitch said, 'floating in a river', can ease stress.

> As we age, a new kind of beauty appears. Every age simply reveals another kind of beautiful.
>
> *Cindy Joseph*
> ....

O

Omega-3

The Australian Menopause Centre writes about the wonders of omega-3 fatty acids and recommends omega-3s as an essential part of a menopausal diet. It has incredible properties for treating a range of menopausal issues. It's been known to assist in:

- reducing the effect of triglycerides to assist in lowering the risk of coronary heart disease
- reducing inflammation, which may help with joint pain and arthritis
- easing the discomfort of the strong menstrual pain and cramping that perimenopausal often experience

- depression—omega-3s work to improve mood and preserve the structural integrity of brain cell membrane health
- osteoporosis—an increased intake of omega-3 acids produces healthier, stronger bones
- hot flushes—studies have shown that while omega-3 may not affect the intensity of hot flushes, it can halve the frequency of hot flushes with the right dosage
- vaginal dryness—a common symptom of menopause, dryness of the vagina can be helped by fatty acids, which help to lubricate the body in general.

How to get enough omega-3 fatty acids

Excellent sources of omega 3 in food:

- oily fish, such as tuna, salmon, herring, sardines and mackerel
- flaxseed and canola oil
- walnuts and walnut oil
- chia seeds
- oysters
- spinach
- soybeans
- eggs
- marine microalgae
- hemp seed oil.

There are also supplements that can give you the Omega 3 that you need.

The Australian National Health and Medical Research Council (NHMRC) suggests a daily intake of 430 micrograms DHA + EPA per day. As this is more than the amount commonly found in a standard fish oil supplement, a good idea for menopausal women is to combine their fish oil supplement with a diet rich in omega-3.[25]

P

Pelvic floor exercises

The onset of menopause can cause your pelvic floor muscles—just like the rest of the muscles in your body—to weaken. These muscles support the pelvic organs, which means that the weakening of these muscles can result in pelvic floor problems.

Pelvic floor muscle exercises are important during this period of a woman's life, and can be beneficial if done correctly. Caution needs to be taken because if the exercises are done incorrectly you can develop pain due to an over-tightened pelvic floor. I personally see a women's health physio who specialises in strengthening and healing the pelvic floor.

Peppermint oil

Peppermint oil is wonderful for fatigue when added to a diffuser, it can calm headaches and help with nausea too. It's been known to assist with cooling off those nights sweats as well. Just be sure to not use it directly on your face, where it can be an irritant.[26]

The trick is to age honestly and gracefully and make it look great, so that everyone looks forward to it.

Emma Thompson
....

Q

Quit smoking

It's well established that premenopausal women who smoke have a significantly higher risk of infertility, difficult menstrual cycles and early menopause, but research over the past few years has established that cigarette smoking also affects menopausal hormones. During the years of the menopausal transition, adding nicotine withdrawal to fluctuating hormones can turn a pussycat into a snarling tiger.

R

Red clover tea

Used primarily to treat hot flushes and night sweats in women with menopause, red clover has also been used to treat high blood pressure, improve bone strength and boost immunity.

Red clover contains phytoestrogens, a plant-based form of oestrogen, which helps to improve the hormonal imbalances caused by menopause. This tea is a delicious way to add red clover to your daily routine. It's important to be aware that if you have breast cancer or have a history of breast cancer, this tea is not for you.[27]

Reiki

As Reiki is known to bring balance to the various systems within the body, it has the ability to bring relief to those suffering from the effects of menopause. Over time, Reiki has been known to normalise menstrual cycles, reduce migraines and cramping, and lessen the frequency of hot flushes. Some women have found Reiki helpful to manage their symptoms. It may be worth looking into. Your health and quality of life should be the central focus of any therapy, and Reiki may be the key to unlocking your ability to heal yourself naturally.

S

Sleep—the cure for what ails you

Three tips to help with the elusive sleep

1. Do whatever you need to do to find the best bed, best mattress, bedding, you name it. Buy it, it's a health investment! We spend so much of our lives in bed, more time than in our fancy cars or designer shoes that you saved years for. So buy exactly the bed you need that will help you to sleep. We need to sleep on the right foundation, no matter what our age. I'm about to buy a cooling pillow, one that apparently stays cool all night and does not heat up from my body. Sounds dreamy.

2. Staying cool in bed is IMPERATIVE. Nothing keeps me awake more than heat at night. So invest in air conditioning. If you can't do that, standing fans can be a life saver. We have one in our bedroom that is silent and amazing. I can angle it right

on me so that Cam is not forming icicles on his head. Cold showers before bed are helpful, lightweight cotton PJs are a must, or nothing at all! Sleep masks can be helpful, as can ear plugs—the more silent and dark the bedroom, the better it is.

3. Be careful what you eat before bed. Obviously caffeine is a killer for a good night's sleep; spicy foods, sugary desserts and alcohol can also be disruptive. Any food with magnesium in it is helpful, such as kiwi fruit, almonds, sesame seeds and bananas. Writing in a journal helps put (some) of my crazy mind to rest at night.

What I've been using

Currently using BioCeuticals MenoPlus 8-PN. I LOVE these pills. They have made a huge difference, especially with my hot flushes at night. I take one in the morning and one at night; they have lavender oil in them so the scent is delightful! And as mentioned elsewhere, lavender works for relaxation in the most lovely subtle way. Bathe in it, sprinkle it on your pillowcase, dab some behind your ears and on your wrists.

I swapped my afternoon caffeine tea for sage tea, and Sleep Superfood Powder by SWIISH is the bomb! It tastes so yummy. I also rub magnesium oil from SWIISH into the souls of my feet. I figure it can't hurt and it's a nice little ritual after my shower to take a little time with my soul (of my feet). (Yes, that was a pun.)

I've stopped having red wine at night. I wish it wasn't the case but after experimenting enough with and without, it's undeniable, red wine makes the hot flushes worse. At least for me.

She stood in the storm, and when the wind did not blow
her way, she adjusted her sails.

Elizabeth Edwards
....

Spiritual and holistic options for general wellbeing

Dr Christiane Northrup is a women's health expert and author
with 25 years' experience as an OB/GYN. She is also an advo-
cate of spiritual and holistic solutions to assist in symptoms of
perimenopause and menopause.[28]

Dr Northrup's suggestions are practical and simple to
integrate into our days. A simple and beautiful routine Dr
Northrup recommends is to take a couple of minutes each
morning and evening by 'revelling in a memory of a time you
felt loved'. Focusing more on loving thoughts will bring about
physical changes that will 'recharge your adrenal batteries'. This
is a way of undoing the harm that stress causes the body. Dr
Northrup encourages us to 'think with our heart' by taking time
out, as a priority rather than a luxury, to focusing on loved ones,
pets, our best traits, our favourite foods and memories, paying
attention to the things in our life that bring us joy and doing
activities that bring us pleasure and make us laugh. That also
means spending less time with people who bring us down and
saying 'no' to those activities that we don't enjoy.

Dr Northrup recommends prioritising—'make a list of your
most important activities and commitments, and then let everything else go'.

Regular light-to-moderate exercise is also high on Dr Northrup's list of helpful activities.

Get more exposure to natural sunlight. It boosts vitamin D and is good for your adrenal glands, as well.

What I've been using

Finding ways to really, wholeheartedly relax has been incredibly rejuvenating. I'm not what I would call a 'meditator'. I'm so sporadic with it, though I've found Deepak Chopra and Oprah Winfrey's 21-day FREE meditation experience truly helpful.[29] There are so many different meditation apps that you can download these days, you'll be sure to find one that works for you.

I need guided meditation, my brain is not programmed (yet) to be able to quiet itself unless someone else is talking me through it. I mean, who doesn't want Oprah's dulcet tones telling me all is well with the world? Some days I would just drift off and have a Nanna Nap, I'm okay with that—having 20 minutes of restful sleep is wonderful for the brain and body and clearly I needed it.

Beware of over-exercising to a point where you are even more exhausted. Exercise can and often is the best remedy for feeling good, but just be mindful of building up to a level that works for you.

I cut back on sugar—lord was (is) that hard. Because I was so tired, my body craved some kind of pick me up, so sugar was waving its arms wildly in the air saying, 'pick me, pick me'. Wrong choice. I fell for this time and time again; I'd have the sugar buzz, feel better for all of 45 minutes, then crash and burn even harder. I found snacking on something that was high in protein gave me the energy to make it through the day. Talking with a dietician about what's right for you and your body is a great step in self-care.

St John's wort

St John's wort is among the most popular herbs used as an alternative treatment for menopausal mood swings, improved sleep, relaxation, and reduced depression and anxiety. Derived from a wild flowering plant called *Hypericum perforatum*, the leaves and flowers are harvested and dried. They can then be brewed in a tea or taken in pill or liquid form.

Scientific studies affirm that while St John's wort is effective for treating mild depression, it works no better than a placebo for treating severe depression.

Make sure to ask your doctor before you begin taking St John's wort, as it might interact with other medications and can have very serious side effects.[30]

Sugar

Is there a connection between sugar and menopause symptoms?

It's been recognised that studies with women who have diets high in sugar can experience worse menopausal symptoms than women with diets low in sugar.

Interestingly, one study that followed 6000 women for nine years found that women who consumed more sugar were 20 per cent more likely to have night sweats and hot flushes. The study showed this was due to, yet again, oestrogen.

Consuming a lot of sugar causes your insulin levels to spike, which simultaneously lowers the amount of a protein in your body called SHBG. SHBG stands for Sex Hormone Binding Globulin, and when your SHBG decreases, your oestrogen goes up. When your oestrogen spikes and falls, your menopausal symptoms worsen.[31]

T

Turmeric

'Turmeric is referred to as "the Golden Goddess" not only for its golden hue and aromatic flavour but also for its healing properties.'[32] Turmeric may assist with pain and fatigue due to the substance curcumin. Turmeric has antioxidant properties that have been said to be great for heart health, hot flushes and depression.

U

Understanding

Knowledge is key when dealing with menopause; be curious about what sets your body off into hot flushes, what bloats you, what eases your spinning mind. Understanding yourself at this time will inevitably help you and gift you with a new sense of yourself.

Unforgiving foods

Added sugars and processed carbs, alcohol and caffeine, spicy foods and high-salt foods. You already know all the bad guys, I'm sure. As a rule, it seems to be: if it tastes really yummy, and you are craving it, it probably means you have to give it up!

My darling girl, when are you going to realise that being normal is not necessarily a virtue? It rather denotes a lack of courage.

Aunt Frances (character), Practical Magic, *Alice Hoffman*

....

V

Vaginal dryness

How to prevent vaginal dryness

You can reduce the risk of vaginal dryness by bringing some changes into your life:

- maintain proper hygiene of your vagina and the area around it
- do not use feminine hygiene products that contain artificial scent
- consider doing Kegel exercises to maintain the elasticity of your vaginal muscles
- always practise safe sex to avoid any sexually transmitted diseases
- consider wearing cotton underwear instead of synthetic underwear—it promotes better airflow and helps your vagina to breathe.

When to see a gynaecologist

Many women feel embarrassed to bring up the topic of vaginal dryness to their doctors. However, it's a severe health condition and can lead to something worse if not treated early.

Over-the-counter lubricants or some home remedies may help reduce the symptoms of vaginal dryness. But if you have other physical issues accompanied by a dry vagina, I suggest seeing your doctor first before consulting your gynaecologist.

Besides, vaginal dryness can have a negative impact on your relationship as it can make sex extremely painful. Hence, it's good to treat this condition as soon as possible.

Home remedies for vaginal dryness

COCONUT OIL

Coconut oil is a popular natural lubricant that you can use for vaginal dryness. It contains linoleic acid, a fatty acid that can deeply moisturise the skin. It can reduce the itchiness, pain, burning and dryness by rejuvenating dry and irritated tissues. Coconut oil can restore the skin's lipid barrier, which helps reduce water loss and aids in strengthening the skin tissues.

Apply extra virgin coconut oil to your vaginal area. Do not mix it with essential oils.

OLIVE OIL

Olive oil is a lipid lubricant that is rich in unsaturated fatty acids. These acids can repair the epithelial tissues in the vagina while keeping it hydrated and moisturised.

In a clinical trial conducted by Australian researchers, 25 women used olive oil as a remedy for vaginal dryness. The oil got a 73 per cent rating in treating this condition.

Olive oil does not cause any side effects, meaning that you can use it without worrying too much.

VITAMIN E OIL

Vitamin E oil can act as a natural lubricant that moisturises your vagina and restores its elasticity. It is a good source of antioxidants that can soothe the irritation and inflammation and provide you with comfort. However, for some women, vitamin E oil may cause irritation and itching. In that case, stop using this oil and consult with your doctor.

JOJOBA OIL

Jojoba oil is rich in essential minerals and vitamins such as vitamin E, vitamin B-complex, copper, zinc, chromium, selenium and iodine.

As jojoba oil is quite gentle, you can use it as a safe alternative to commercial lubricant for the vagina. The moisturising components in jojoba oil can mimic the sebum on your skin, meaning that it can effectively treat vaginal dryness.

EVENING PRIMROSE OIL

Evening primrose oil originates from the seeds of the evening primrose plant through cold pressing. The oil is commonly used to treat various skin disorders such as eczema, psoriasis, and acne.

PHYTOESTROGEN-RICH DIET

Vaginal dryness can occur if the oestrogen level is reduced. A diet rich in phytoestrogen can help you alleviate this problem. Phytoestrogen is a plant-based oestrogen that can balance the hormone levels in your body. Besides, it can lubricate your vagina by producing more oestrogens. It can also improve libido in postmenopausal women.

You can include phytoestrogen-rich food, such as carrots, barley, cherries, flaxseeds and licorice root, in your daily diet to reduce vaginal dryness.[33]

Women with breast cancer or who have a history of breast cancer should seek medical advice before adopting a phytoestrogen-rich diet.

OVER-THE-COUNTER LUBE

A lot of books and websites recommend buying lubricant. Make sure it is water-based as the silicon ones can sometimes have a negative effect on the sensitive area of your vagina.

W

Water

During menopause, women often experience dryness. This is likely caused by the decrease in oestrogen levels. Water is critical for menopausal women to hydrate cells, moisturise skin, and eliminate toxins from the body. Try to get at least six cups a day. If you measure it into a large bottle or pitcher at the beginning of the day, you can see your progress and try to finish it up by bedtime.

I am proud of the woman I am today, I went through one hell of a time to become her.

@pelvicpainhelp
....

X

Xany

(adj) wild; overly energetic
This may just be the new you. A wildness that emerges.

Xenacious

(adj) yearning for change
Changes are happening within us; maybe you need to make some changes to your lifestyle, relationships or career—let the yearning change your course.

Xoompin

(v) to drive over bumps on the road
Well, have we not done a whole lot of xoompin? Bumps, potholes, gosh darn cliffs, we've navigated so much. You are officially an expert driver of *you*.

Y

Yoga

Yoga is well known for relieving stress. A few studies have found that yoga, tai chi and similar mind—body therapies may also improve certain menopausal symptoms, such as sleeping issues and hot flush, in some women.

So how can yoga help women during menopause?

- It lowers stress. Yoga controls breathing, which in turn reduces anxiety. It also clears all the negative feelings and thoughts from the mind, leading to the reduction of depression. It is a proven, effective method to reduce and control anger. When practising yoga regularly the overall sense of calmness increases and as a result a happier, stress-free life can be led.

- It eases physical pain and discomfort. Yoga practitioners are known to have higher pain tolerance. Aches and pains associated with menopause can be eased along with any back pain, chronic pain or neck pain you may be experiencing. A gentle practice of the flowing Surya Namaskar (sun salutation) helps to increase flexibility in the joints and works every muscle in the body, a complete physical and emotional workout in itself. Try practising five to ten rounds per day; even if you don't have time for other yoga you will experience dramatic relief from general aches and pains.

- It decreases the hassles of hot flushes. During menopause, hot flushes are caused by an excess of *pitta* (fire) in the body and that has to come out! General asanas (yoga postures) that help with this include *ardha baddha padma paschimottanasana* (half-bound lotus pose), *ardha matsyendrasana* (half lord of the fishes pose) and *supta padmasana* (reclined or sleeping lotus pose). Movements should be slow and weight bearing, paying close attention to the rhythm of the breath and position of the tongue to the roof of the palate during practice. This allows the mind to become calm and stabilise.

- It reduces blood pressure. A common symptom during the menopause is night sweats. Regular yoga practice reduces high blood pressure and promotes oxygenation and blood circulation in the body, in turn easing the terrible night sweats. *Shavasana* (corpse pose) is perfect for allowing yourself to relax and just bring your attention to the breath. By taking your focus away from the stresses and strains of the outside world, you focus on what's happening now and on managing any anxieties.

- It's a natural remedy. Yoga is a fantastic and natural way to help alleviate pain. So many women suffer in silence, or take endless pills, but yoga is an ideal way to soothe hormonal symptoms, that you can do either in a group or in the comfort of your own home. It helps bring you to a calmer place emotionally and physically.

- It's even better when combined with aromatherapy. Yoga and aromatherapy have physical, mental and spiritual benefits for the practitioner and therefore it becomes logical to use aromatherapy when practising yoga. Not only are your senses enthralled by the beautiful aromas during your practice, the focus and effects of your practice are intensified by the therapeutic use of the essential oil blends. Healing benefits of aromatherapy oils include releasing old or negative emotions, experiencing a detoxifying or cleansing feeling, soothing tense muscles, helping to balance hormonal fluctuations or even helping to realign the chakras and promote feelings of calm and peace.

- It's great for the joints. Yoga has been proven to help people suffering from problems associated with joints, such as arthritis. While not all menopausal women will have arthritis, it's a health concern that's often associated with ageing. Research from the United States shows that practicing hatha yoga can help to ease joint pain, fatigue and other related symptoms. The small study involved women aged 21 to 35 who, on average, had suffered from rheumatoid arthritis for ten and a half years. After six weeks, they asked both groups about their condition. The group that practised yoga said they were happier than when they started and could better accept and manage their pain. The women were also reported to have better general health and more energy in general.[34]

Z

Zinc

Magdalena Wszelaki writes on the website hormonesbalance.com that zinc is an essential trace element that's found in and used by every cell throughout your body. Anytime a nutrient is considered 'essential' it means your body needs it to stay healthy but that you can't produce it and therefore you must get it from your food.

This critical metal is only needed in tiny amounts but if you don't get enough zinc, the consequences can be grave. This is because your body relies on zinc for growth, maintenance and numerous biological functions—including hormone creation and balance. Zinc's impact on your hormones is a big deal.

First of all, you need sufficient levels of zinc for your body to create hormones. Then you also need sufficient zinc to maintain a proper hormonal balance.

Here are the top fifteen best food sources of zinc:

1. oysters
2. grass-fed beef
3. turkey breast
4. lamb
5. sesame seeds
6. pasture-raised chicken
7. beans
8. pumpkin seeds
9. peanuts
10. cashews
11. sunflower seeds
12. cocoa
13. pork
14. egg
15. almonds.[35]

Zizyphus

The fruit of the zizyphus tree is used as food and to make medicine. It is most admired and used for its effective treatment of sleep conditions, such as insomnia, nervous exhaustion, night sweats, palpitations and excessive perspiration. Traditionally it is prescribed for people experiencing restless sleep, troubling dreams, anxiety and even concentration problems.[36]

CHAPTER 10

Magical powers of
menopause

According to a survey commissioned by *Health Plus* magazine, 72 per cent of postmenopausal women think they are 'just as attractive as before', 82 per cent feel 'as feminine as before', 80 per cent feel an 'overwhelming sense of freedom', and 60 per cent feel 'better than ever before'.[1] More good news: the average postmenopausal woman feels ten years younger than her real age.

> Some research shows that around 50 percent of women report being happiest and most fulfilled between the ages of 50 and 65 compared with when they were in their 20s, 30s or 40s.[2]
>
> *Dr Axe*
> ....

As I write this book, I realise that my curiosity isn't all down to menopause, it's down to the miraculous ability of women to adapt and change, to walk through the fire and come out the other side changed, brighter and better. What *is* this midlife challenge we are all headed towards or going through? Menopause is a part of it, absolutely. But this movement within wakes us up, shakes us to our bones and whispers in our ear: get up and *do* something. We may not know what. I know I didn't know 'what', but following that feeling, that feeling of 'the change' and directing it towards a goal, a desire, is a long-held dream. That's the midlife that I want, the one I want you all to have.

So, let's knock out a list here. Let's find that silver lining, because it's there—sometimes you just need to put your new glasses on to see it.

Here we go:

1. No more 'Am I pregnant?' or 'Where are the condoms?' moments, no more being on the pill or withdrawal method needed.

     You can literally have sex anywhere, anytime, anyplace. Will you? Maybe not, but the magical powers of menopause grant you the gift of being able to. Or fantasising about it. Or talking about it with your girlfriends, at least. Many women feel way more sexually liberated after menopause.

     After menopause our progesterone and oestrogen decrease, but guess what hangs around a bit more? Mr Testosterone, and so with the balance of testosterone leading the way, your sex drive might just be on the up and up. I know, it's possible you will experience vaginal dryness and painful sex, but not everyone has these symptoms, and if you do, don't stress—there are lubricants for that and you can get imaginative with your love life. After the same routine sex with the same partner, maybe changing things up could be just the treat your sex life needs.

2. No more wondering when I'll bleed, no more embarrassing leaks or jumpers tied around the waist in the middle of winter, no more realising that you don't actually have a spare tampon/ pad in your purse like you thought so will have to make do with a public restroom rolled-up bunch of toilet paper shoved into your underwear that invariably moves around and keeps you dry for all of two minutes. No more I can't swim today on the first day of your period when you feel you may attract a small school of sharks if you enter the water. No more spending money on sanitary products or chucking out your favourite pair of underwear because you can't get the bloodstain out. No more adding to landfill by using sanitary products—you are a newborn eco warrior. You are *saving* the *environment*! No more buying bleach and spot remover for your gorgeous 1400-count Egyptian sheets. Presto, done.

3. You might just be the healthiest you that you've ever been. Menopause could be a wake-up call to become kinder and healthier with our bodies. It certainly forced me to make changes that before perimenopause I was simply avoiding: eating cleaner, exercising, meditating, being diligent with my

vitamins, and creating a better sleep schedule have all happened due to the magical powers of menopause. As I've mentioned multiple times in the book, self-care is of utmost importance.

Putting energy into creating special time and care for yourself is a delightful treat. Putting yourself in the number one spot on your to-do list might feel weird at first, but you deserve it. Honestly, without the crazy symptoms of menopause, I believe I would have continued down the path of a very unhealthy life.

4. You can break free from the belief system that beauty is only for the young, let go of the expectation that we as women need to remain young and youthful to be relevant. Whose approval are we seeking? You can now let go of all the societal 'shoulds' and examine what it is you actually want for yourself. Menopause does not define you; you define who you are, at any age and at any time. We are being called to live more authentically, to connect with what our heart desires. Allowing menopause to shift your outlook to positive may be challenging, but the outcome is nothing short of magical.

5. Creatively, we are also on fire, and I don't mean with our hot flushes. Our uterus is where we create life, literally. When we are no longer fertile enough to carry a child, we have the energy to redirect our creativity toward other uses. I've seen and heard this over and over again: redirecting your creativity into something you love may change your career path or enlighten the one you are already on, or simply give you a damn fun hobby that you will love. We can be overflowing

with creativity. Magically we are less afraid to fail, so start using that creative energy for something you love.

6. This might just be a time to take stock of your life, and what you've accomplished. Write it down, write *everything* down, from the sweet successes to the smallest of positives (I finally learned how to make the perfect quiche). With all that you've learned and the knowledge you have gained, what's next? Recognising how far you've come in your life and what you've needed to work through to not only survive but thrive is a great way to move forward with your life. Look back at everything you have done. Pat your self on the back and keep making plans to conquer the world.

7. Knowing someone is an arsehole before they even speak. Your intuition is strong, you've seen enough bullshit in your life to know the difference between fake and genuine. You spend your time with the people who are your tribe and don't sweat over the ones you don't like anyway. This is a gooooooood superpower. As you're no longer willing to put up with crap from other people, the friends you now surround yourself with will most likely be the ones who will carry you through the rest of your life. You've done the sorting and found the gems.

8. Self-belief is a superpower and from what I've seen from women in their fifties and beyond, there is a belief in themselves that is undeniable. That can only come from living

through some heavy experiences and coming through the other side victorious. We've grown through some tough times by now, and maybe there are more ahead, though with everything you've learned along the way, your armoury of tools to deal with it all is immense.

9. When our focus is on who moves us, and who cares, listens to and understands us, the connections to others become so much deeper and richer.

10. Choosing moisturisers becomes easy. Instead of needing different creams for skin texture variations, there's only dry, dry, and more dry. I can slather oils on my face till the cows come home and my skin laps it up with delight.

11. I am almost never cold. I am basically my own furnace that can shelter my children from arctic blasts of wind and keep the roast chicken warm in my armpits if needed to. I am a human oven.

12. Having been someone who felt lonely for much of my life, I've noticed that those feelings are gone. Having time alone is now not only comfortable, but healing and necessary. I'm so grateful to finally feel comfortable enough in my own skin to be alone.

13. Okay, stay with me here, it's a doozy. You are like an *orca whale*, that's right, an orca. There are only three animals that experience menopause: humans, pilot whales and orcas.

I mean, I love pilot whales too, but orcas? Super cool, let me explain. Female orcas reach menopause around 30 to 40 years old. Why? According to *National Geographic*:

One of the most compelling explanations is called the grand-mother hypothesis. Proposed in 1966, it suggests that older females forgo the option to bear more children so they can support their existing ones. By helping their children and grandchildren to survive and thrive, they still ensure that their genes cascade down the generations.[3]

So when anyone asks you if you are going through 'the change', you can say, 'Why yes, I am becoming an orca whale and leading my pod,' or something like that—but much more funny and interesting. I was trying to come up with a *Free Willy* reference but just didn't find one good enough.

14. Uterine fibroids shrink. Many women approaching their fifties develop fibroids, uterine tumours that are almost always benign. Fibroids grow when oestrogen levels in the body are high, but fibroids often stop growing or shrink when women reach menopause and oestrogen levels decline. For women who have fibroids sitting on their bladder, meno-pause can give them a break!

15. Menopause can help endometriosis. While it's not proven that every woman with endometriosis will be relieved of the pain they experience once menopause hits, for many women, when

menstruation stops, the symptoms related to endometriosis will lessen somewhat.

16. I feel mature enough to understand that when I feel down I should not trust the way I see myself. Learning to love myself, even when I feel less than whole, has been one of the biggest lessons of my life so far. Menopause has pushed me to the very edge of that truth. Can I love myself in *all* the places where I feel I am crumbling, aging, changing? The answer is simple, because what other choice is there? Yes, yes, I can love myself in every place. Why wouldn't I? I would do the same for my children, husband, another family member or friend. May we all pour love on all the places we have felt ugly and lost and afraid. Flood the hatred and judgement with kindness.

A woman is the full circle. Within her is the power to create, nurture and transform.

Diane Mariechild
....

Things I know about healing: speaking kindly to yourself helps. A lot.

Rebecca Ray
....

Journal entry, October 2019

Something shifted. The hot flushes are coming rarely now, only maybe two a night at most. Sleep still eludes me, though I don't feel as exhausted. I feel a new sort of energy, in fact. A creative energy. I want to paint, make pottery, write a novel. I want to travel and learn another language. I want to be more daring and colourful with how I dress. I want to create a better, more physically intimate relationship with my husband—I don't know what that looks like, but I finally feel ready.

You will learn a lot about yourself if you stretch in the direction of goodness, of bigness, of kindness, of forgiveness, of emotional bravery. Be a warrior for love.

Cheryl Strayed
·················

CHAPTER 11

Postmenopause

Let's hear from some well-known women who are not only successful, but intelligent, kind and gorgeous.

It's easy to believe that celebrities have it better, but trust me, celebrities are exactly the same as everyone else—they just have to go through menopause publicly.

Each of these women has generously shared their story of menopause with me, in the hope you don't feel so alone. So you may know that menopause is not a life-ender, but a life-changer . . . and for the BETTER!

As the wonderful Brené Brown says, 'When we deny our stories, they define us. When we own our stories, we get to write a brave new ending.'[1]

Own your story, share your story and write your ending. May it be the most funky, fabulous, luscious, joyful ending ever.

Georgie Parker

Georgie is one of Australia's most beloved actresses. She has appeared in multiple TV series, films and theatre productions; she has won the coveted Gold Logie twice, and more recently she has appeared on and hosted the successful *The All New Monty: Ladies' Night* show, which raised awareness around testicular and breast cancer. When I was looking for women who might be willing to share their post-menopause story, Georgie was quick to offer her support. She is one generous and kind lady. Georgie shares with us her experience of being on HRT and how it has worked positively for her.

When I was eighteen/nineteen my mum went through menopause and it was very debilitating for her. Her mood was inconsistent and unpredictable and her volcanic hot flushes were very distressing for her. She would saturate her clothes through and change colour. These happened day and night.

I started going through perimenopause at exactly the same age as my mum, 49 years old, and I swiftly went straight into menopause.

To try and deal with my symptoms, which were predominantly hot (volcanic) flushes, I tried a type of antidepressant (a side effect of which is that it can treat and manage heat), then I tried a synthetic hormone, and I tried Happy Hormones, teas, herbal treatments and remedies, a change of diet, etc. Some things worked for two months then stopped working completely; some didn't work at all.

The biggest change for me is I don't get my period anymore—rejoice. And my sexual drive and energy are more intermittent—there is no way around that. But apart from that I feel great, actually.

My friends do all talk about menopause and the impact it's had on our lives and our relationship to ourselves and others. A woman's body is required to do so much; it's built for it, designed for it, but the cost of these constant changes can be difficult to process.

The judgement and expectations we put on ourselves don't help. Some of my mates find menopause discombobulating and with other women it has no impact. Isn't it strange!

I went on HRT, like my mother, to deal with the lack of sleep and trying to work fourteen-hour days. The lack of sleep was worse than when I had a newborn, and waking up in a saturated mess every 40 minutes was not something I was prepared to put myself through. So after seven months of trying other things I ventured into my HRT experience and it's been amazing. I literally have nothing but positive things to say about it.

I have talked with Steve (my husband) a lot over the years about my menopause and symptoms, but I'm very independent when it comes to my physical wellbeing, a result of having to deal with scoliosis since I was thirteen, I suspect. He's been supportive, of course, but it is my journey and I like to deal with it in my own way and be in my headspace with it. He's always up for a big conversation though, so if I need him, he's there.

I have to say, menopause has been exactly what I thought it would be: difficult. But once I committed to a treatment plan, it's been much more manageable. I've gone exactly the way my mum did, minus the emotional component, thank God.

My view, idea or concept of my femininity hasn't really changed, but it's shifted, and I love that. I no longer have the clock of ovulation to mark my life by. I feel much freer, I feel strong and I feel in control. I still feel connected to my sexual energy even though I literally don't feel like sharing it that regularly.

The interesting time will be when I go off HRT. I'm slowly lowering my dose so I'm on four pills a week rather than seven, and I'll keep playing with that till I'm off.

My advice to other women? Wow, it's such a personal 'event', so to speak. I loath to suggest there's a right or wrong way. But explore your options, and if you're going through a fresh kind of hell, seek medical advice—it varies greatly. If you're happy to grit your teeth and get through it, that's great, too. Find YOUR happy place, that's my advice.

Sally Obermeder

Sally's list of credentials is long and varied. She's a TV presenter, journalist, radio host, best-selling author and, with her sister Maha, heads up the hugely successful SWIISH—a wellness and lifestyle brand. Sally was diagnosed with an aggressive form of breast cancer the day before she gave birth to her first child, Annabelle Grace, in 2011. She underwent eleven months of gruel-ling chemotherapy and a double mastectomy, and successfully beat it. This did, however, caused early menopause. Sally has used her experience to maintain the most beautiful and positive outlook on life, becoming a beacon of hope and inspiration to us all.

I remember Mum talking about menopause. I remember it in a negative context. I remember her saying to my dad, 'I'm not having HRT. My doctor is trying to force me to have HRT and I don't want it, I'm worried about it giving me cancer.' She wanted to take a natural approach so she got onto Remifemin. It was the first time I'd ever heard of that. That was it, no discussion around what she was feeling, what she was going through—it was her versus the doctor and she felt she wasn't being heard. She kept what she was going through very quiet.

My menopause was medically induced. I did so much chemo due to cancer. I was 38, and I was right on the cusp of sliding into menopause. I really didn't want to. I didn't want anything else to happen to my body. I had already been through so much. I was holding out and it was a case of wait and see if my period comes back. I finished all my treatments, and I waited.

I was so excited when I did get my period, I bawled my eyes out. I said to my husband, Marcus, 'The most amazing thing just happened, I just got my period.' In a way I equated me getting my period back as my body healing, functioning. I placed a lot of weight on that. Tick, I am whole again.

Periods were choppy for four or five months, then they never came back. My doctor did a blood test and that was it, I was in menopause. I was so sad, I already knew I couldn't carry a child, but this seemed like a death, like a part of my body had died.

Everyone around me was still quite young and nobody was going through menopause and I felt quite alone. I wasn't sure who to speak with about this, so I didn't really say anything to anyone. I just sucked it up. Didn't want to be any trouble.

Menopause still has a 'yucky' vibe about it that it doesn't need to, but it does. It has a death vibe about it, but not in a way where anyone lets you say, okay, I'm mourning the end of this chapter and it's also the beginning of another chapter. So then you just stay quiet.

It was a funny time. For a little less than a year I didn't really have any symptoms. I also think my body was still recovering from all the chemo. Once my body started to find its equilibrium again, then I started to get night sweats. I'd say to Marcus, 'There is something wrong with the mattress. I think it's on fire.' My body felt like it was literally on fire. I don't know if I was any more or less moody. Because I had gone through cancer, it changes your mindset, so deeply. There is a real gratitude about simply being alive. I was on a real mission to have another baby via a surrogate, so I had something to focus on that kept my mood really up. My skin became paper thin and dry; no matter how much I moisturised, it was always dry until I started taking collagen. Lack of sexual desire, so weird, what is going on? My body was changing.

What helped me was my mindset—knowing you are in for the ride. I'm just going to give in, I'd rather be alive with menopause than the other option. I'm going to go with the flow. I'm not going to beat myself up over anything. If I feel shitty, I feel shitty. I now eat better than I used to. I slept more to recover better. I don't sweat the small stuff.

HRT was not an option for me; there was nothing for me to have as a hormonal option. That's what got me started working on a natural hormone replacement with SWIISH. If you can't have HRT you need something natural.

The biggest change for me is that proverbial line in the sand where I don't feel young. Menopause is like, this is you before, and okay now you are in the second half of your life and you can't go back. I had to wrap my head around that. It's an internal shift. We are now in this phase. I'm with the older people now, I've crossed over. I went from zero to 100, as I had no perimenopause. It was a lot. I thought I'd get my period back, my health, and be able to have another baby. It was as if while I slept someone just closed up the shop.

The positive changes I've experienced now I'm in menopause are that now I know I can't please everyone. I've stopped trying. I realised I don't have 80 years ahead of me. This is what I want to do, this is how I want to live, these are the toxic people I'm ejecting from my life, this is what makes me happy, this is what I need, this is what I want to give, this is my purpose. I don't have time to fuck around. I want to live my life the way I see fit. I trust my gut so much more. This is what's right, what feels right. The whispers in the ear are drowned out; I trust my heart and my gut so much more. You can't please everyone.

My advice to any woman, especially any woman who is headed into medically induced menopause, is: don't be afraid and don't be ashamed—it's nothing to feel inferior about—you are still awesome. And speak up. We don't speak up enough. No one ever speaks about menopause

When I had trouble conceiving, I didn't use IVF at first because I didn't speak up enough about it, so I waited. I just thought I had a faulty body. Everyone else seemed to be having a baby at the drop of a hat. But we've had a real shift in talking about IVF and fertility. I would like to see the same shift around menopause. Why is menopause in the closet, so to speak? It shouldn't be. It's not weird or bad, it's just a phase. Like the way we talk about puberty, having children. It should be as easy to speak about as anything to do with fertility and reproduction.

Lynne McGranger

I had the best conversation with Lynne as she was making her way to the set of *Home and Away*. We chatted for a long time. Lynne was so honest, funny and generous with her story; she is a great example of how women telling stories about menopause is a powerful tool. Lynne is most well known for her role in the iconic Aussie soap. She has starred as Irene Roberts for 30 years, which is clearly a testament to how important Lynne is to the show. In 2014 she was acknowledged as a TV actor legend when she became the longest-serving female cast member of any Australian TV show. She has also received critical acclaim for her stage roles in Harold Pinter's *The Lover*, and *Honey*, an award-winning play based on Bryce Courtenay's *Smoky Joe's Cafe*. She is an Australian national treasure.

The first time I understood anything about menopause was when I was thirteen and my mum was 42 and she needed to go to hospital for a hysterectomy. She went through early menopause. My mum was a fairly calm sort of person. I remember her getting a bit tetchy with Dad, which was out of character. So when I spoke with her when I was an adult and menopause was looming for me, I asked her about it. It wasn't really a big deal for her. I don't even think she took anything for her hormones. Mum was as fit as a mallee bull and she just got on with it.

Because my mother seemingly swept through menopause so easily, I didn't really worry. I felt I didn't really need any advice from her as it was a non-event.

The first change I noticed was around age 49/50. I remember this period that would not go away—it lasted for about three weeks. I'd never been very regular and I'd never had very heavy periods either. (Getting pregnant so easily was probably a bit of a miracle.) I figured it was the start of menopause.

So I went to see my doctor and she gave me these 'horse tablets', which I'm assuming were either progesterone or oestrogen. I was told to just take one a day till my period stops and after about a week it stopped and that was it. I never had it again.

I stopped taking the tablets and just got on with it.

I do remember taking Remifemin for a while in combination with MenoEze, which the famous actress Rowena Wallace used to advertise. Hot drinks and alcohol were something I stayed away from.

I did have the hot flushes that felt volcanic, that started in the pit of my belly and then gradually bubbled up and like a cartoon character. I felt like my head was going to explode. But I didn't have them for a long time and gradually they decreased in intensity and frequency and over a period of a year they went away. Now I have no hot flushes at all.

My changes were more about lack of libido and a dryness in my vagina and getting pernickety with my partner, or possibly he was just giving me the shits!

I guess I was a bit hormonal with him.

Coffee and hairdryers were anathema to me.

Of course, working on the TV show *Home and Away*, first thing in the morning, coffee and hairdryers were par for the course. The hot flushes back then were a bit embarrassing. I'd be sitting in a group somewhere and a wave of heat would overwhelm me.

I do remember a time, thinking back now about fifteen years ago, when my relationship with my partner was quite fractured and my father was dying and I was quite depressed. I thought it was more about not being on the same page as my partner. I was trying to give up smoking and many things were crashing in on me. Now I realise that menopause could very well have been an issue—I didn't realise it at the time. I do think my feelings were exaggerated because of my hormones. I was very close to leaving my partner, certainly our communication broke down. So menopause may have ramped it up.

I didn't talk about menopause much with my partner, to be honest, and this is interesting to me; I probably was a bit embarrassed by it, which is peculiar, because it's like being embarrassed about getting your period or having a baby or breastfeeding—it's part of the natural cycle of life. But I guess looking back on it, I felt it was kind of admitting I was getting old and was no longer attractive and sexy—maybe that's what it was for me. I still wanted to be this youngish attractive person that my partner fell in love with.

But it is what it is, and like any form of getting older, men age, too; he has his beer belly and all the changes for him when you hit 60. We never dwelled on it. When it came to sex, we made amends, even though the dry vagina was real. Maybe it is nature's way of telling you to stop having sex. But there are ways and means and there are helpful products.

I didn't really speak about menopause or joke about it. I really admired the women who did. I'm the first person to have a joke about anything inappropriate, I just didn't really speak about menopause.

It was me admitting I was getting old.

My sexuality changed; my libido didn't completely disappear, and it's good that you are no longer the 'root rat' that you were in your thirties! Other things become much more important. I'm very much comfortable in my own skin. I feel fit for my age and healthy for my age.

I just need to keep my memory and brain in good condition.

I exercise a lot, which I find keeps me in great stead, and this helps with not only my physical shape but my mental shape as well.

When I have periods of forgetfulness and I can't think of something, I use a trick that works 95 per cent of the time: I go through the alphabet. I won't google. I'll dig through the recesses of my brain and I almost always get it. I do brain games as well, code words to keep my brain sharp. I read a lot and keep my brain active.

I saw my mum lose confidence when she would be forgetful, so I work on my short-term memory.

Don't let menopause define you and, if you start to lose your libido, do what I didn't do and discuss it with your partner and come up with ways that could counteract the loss of physical intimacy. It does involve your partner. I'd suggest seeing a naturopath or a kinesiologist to address the issues before they become too big. Talk to your girlfriends, too, in a way I wish I'd done. My closest group of friends were just not the same age as me, so they were not going through it when I was. Talk about it more. Having said that, menopause never really affected me badly.

Anita Heiss

Anita is a proud member of the Wiradjuri nation of central New South Wales, and is one of Australia's most prolific and well-known authors, publishing across genres, including non-fiction, historical fiction, commercial fiction and children's novels.

Anita is proud to be a Lifetime Ambassador for the Indigenous Literacy Foundation, and an Ambassador of Worawa Aboriginal College, the GO Foundation and the Sydney Swans.

She is on the Board of University of Queensland Press and Circa Contemporary Circus, and is a Professor of Communications at the University of Queensland.

With La Boite Theatre, she is currently adapting her novel *Tiddas* for the stage.

Anita is quite frankly a powerhouse. To quote her, she 'firmly believes that sharing stories to build respect can connect us as humans.'

I couldn't agree more.

Menopause is like puberty for adults

NADINE: I know it's not an excuse, but I'm sick. [The *tiddas* look concerned. IZZY rests her hand on NADINE's]

IZZY: What is it?

NADINE: Menopause.

ELLEN: Oh for fuck's sake, Nadine [rolls eyes]. Menopause isn't a fucking illness, it's a fucking life cycle, like puberty for grown-ups.

NADINE: Thanks for the sympathy, Ellen; you'll feel differently as soon as you start getting the symptoms. I know you think everything I say is 'white race privilege' but I tell you, menopause does not discriminate by race, age or socioeconomics.

By Anita Heiss

This scene is from the stage adaption of my novel *Tiddas*[2] and it was borne out of a conversation with a guy I once dated. He advised me that his ex-wife was very sick, and when I enquired with concern what the illness was, imagining it to be something horrific like cancer, he responded seriously with, 'Menopause! She's going to go on HRT.'

I didn't laugh at the time, but wish now I had, because Ellen's response above is how I feel about menopause; it is part of the life cycle, like puberty for adults.

There is so little research on Aboriginal women and menopause that it isn't worth mentioning. Perhaps it's because we are forced to be resilient at a very young age; perhaps we complain less than our non-Indigenous counterparts when other things in life are far more important to discuss, or perhaps we see the change of life as just that, a change, a process, a reality that is something we simply endure like everything else in life. Perhaps we just aren't that quick to swallow Western medicine either. I mean, we managed without it for tens of thousands of years, didn't we?

I confess that at 52 years of age, there's not a lot I am sure about on the menopause front. I'd like to say that I am through menopause, but who knows? The symptoms come and go, and the joys of this change of life include the uncertainty of an end date.

I don't remember when the hot flushes started, but back in August of 2016, when I had night sweats in the middle of winter while I was visiting Melbourne, I knew I could no longer blame the Brisbane humidity for ruining my sleep. It had to be menopause, or perimenopause at least, because I was still getting my period. I was just on 48 years old, and I'd been feeling the impact of 'the change' for at least six months.

I recall going to my GP upon returning from the Melbourne Writers Festival and advising him that I was in fact perimenopausal (clearly my PhD in Communication and Media gave me some knowledge in medicine as well). He sent me for blood tests only to advise soon after that my oestrogen levels were still too high for me to be menopausal. He then proceeded to lecture me on safe sex and the possibility of me still falling pregnant.

'STOP! Please stop,' I implored. 'This conversation is not necessary.' At that age I did not need a lesson on safe sex or advice on contraception.

I went home, started taking Promensil and Femular Forte, which are herbal remedies that assist with hot flushes, night sweats, insomnia and other symptoms. I took them hopefully and regularly and tried to sleep—doona on, doona off, doona on again, with the ceiling fan spinning all year round. The doctor may have been thrown off by the test results, but I certainly wasn't. And nor was my body.

I never contemplated HRT as a real tool for dealing with the symptoms of menopause. The side effects concerned me—and I pretty much had enough going on without changes to my body to add to them. But, after the most painful pap smear of my life left me shaken and in tears, and at my new lady doctor's advice, I decided to try an oestrogen pessary to assist with lessening potentially painful sex in the future, because what I wasn't prepared for was being a virtual born-again virgin! But for the few weeks I used the pessary I was constantly nauseous, and when I worked out what was causing the nausea I stopped. No promise of painless sex was worth feeling ill all day for.

So, I am not on HRT, but occasionally I still reach for Promensil or Femular. I haven't had a period in 2020 but I still suffer with interrupted sleep. I still have hot flushes (or flashes as they say in the United States) and I'm still blaming my unshiftable stomach fat on 'menopausal hormones'.

It's fair to say I was not expecting anything in particular in terms of going into menopause. I'd never really given it more than a fleeting thought. From memory my mother didn't talk about it, and neither do many of my friends. I do recall a couple of brief conversations with one or two girlfriends suggesting they might kill their husbands if they did not have HRT because their behaviour had become irrational and at times uncontrollable. I didn't really understand their emotions back then. At one appointment, though, I did tell my doctor that I was so tired I was going to throw a chair at someone if I didn't get some decent sleep. Since then, melatonin has become a friend when needed.

The thought of hitting menopause never concerned me. In fact, all I could think about and look forward to was no more period! The inconvenience and expense, to say nothing of the bloating and pain associated with a woman's monthly cycle, well, menopause had to be better than that. Never being maternal, menopause for me meant freedom. So it was surprising to me to hear other women feel sad about entering this phase of their life. To some it meant that they would never have their first, or another, child. I'd never thought about menopause that way.

In all honesty, until recently, my friends never discussed menopause much, and certainly not my Aboriginal friends. I seem to talk about it more than anyone I know, and a couple of Aboriginal tiddas have asked me for advice, because they, too, don't have many friends who discuss it. It makes me wonder if we as Aboriginal women are just used to getting on with it. Not complaining about the inevitable, about what is natural.

I remember sitting with a group of Murri women in Brisbane when I was researching my novel *Tiddas*. I was writing about Nadine—the character mentioned before—and those women mentioned kangaroo as a way of managing menopause. I had long eaten roo without knowing that.

As I write this, I think about my sense of womanhood, my sense of self and femininity, and I can honestly say I have never felt better about myself as a woman. I feel healthy, I feel in control of my body, and my self-esteem is the best it has ever been (but I have struggled with body image since childhood).

For the women who have menopause to look forward to, I need to tell you that your body will do things you will not like. In no particular order:

- Your belly will increase regardless of exercise and diet, and you will be disappointed when nothing you do changes it. Trust me, I run three times a week, I do PT; if I lose weight it comes off my knees before my gut. That's menopause.
- Your vagina will dry up, literally. Sex will hurt, pap smears will hurt. You will need to find ways to make things 'fit'. That's menopause.
- The hot flushes may leave your entire body in millions of beads of sweat without warning, day and night. You may be in a fancy restaurant in your favourite black dress only to have huge drops of sweat fall from your body. That's menopause. [Tip: always keep a fan in your handbag!]

There is no shame in talking about menopause. It is part of being a woman, and being a woman is wonderful, most days. So, talk about it if you need to, and do what you need to do to get through what might take years to be complete. But understand that women the world over have coped, and continue to 'cope', with this stage of life without chemicals, without drama and without thinking you have an 'illness'.

Rhonda Burchmore

Rhonda is known lovingly as 'Australia's Leading Lady'. Her career has spanned over 35 years in the entertainment industry, and she is immensely popular and beloved by her peers. Her theatre credits range from *Sugar Babies* in the West End to *Into the Woods*, *Urinetown* and so many more. She has also gone on to write and produce successful shows. She is regularly seen on TV as well as singing her heart out on Australian morning television. In 2014 Rhonda was awarded the OAM for her service to the performing arts and community.

Rhonda has recorded five albums, including *Pure Imagination*, *Midnight Rendezvous*, *Live at the Melbourne Concert Hall* and *Cry Me A River: The World of Julie London* with ABC Records. Rhonda's story is fabulous, as she breezed through menopause. It's an important story to let women know that there are many women whose symptoms are barely a blip!

Growing up, my mother Yvonne was extremely conservative and never spoke about anything to do with menopause. In fact, my mother never even had 'the talk' with me about puberty. I gather she just expected that I would find out about it from school 'personal development classes' and talking with my friends. She bordered on embarrassed if the subject was even brought up.

I noticed the first signs of perimenopause at around 50 years old when I started to develop extremely heavy periods and cramping but nothing else significant. When I was mid-fifties I started to notice a little thinning of my hair on the right side of my head, I wasn't sure whether this was related to menopause or just aging.

I never felt the need to take any medicine or remedies. There was nothing that extreme that couldn't be fixed with extra protection for any period leaks and Nurofen Plus.

The best and most positive thing about my menopause is the fact that I no longer need to worry about that 'time of the month', going out on stage or in public with the fear of extreme bleeding and cramping. It was a nightmare for a while due to the unpredictability of it all. I would be forced to use super-strength tampons and pads, which were often uncomfortable. I certainly do not miss all of that.

I have touched on menopause when talking with my friends. We'd discuss it—only as a light topic though. It seems compared to some of my friends I got off lightly!

My partner was of course aware when I was going through menopause, but because it was pretty uneventful we didn't really discuss it much.

Menopause has been much easier than I expected. I never experienced a lot of the symptoms others do, including mood swings and night sweats, etc.

I've not felt my femininity shift or change. I just accept that I am getting older, and everyone will at some stage so it's a natural part of life.

My advice to women who have yet to reach this point in their life is to not stress—feel comfortable to talk to your friends about it and know that what you're experiencing is normal. As a mother of a daughter I freely encourage discussion about all things to do with our bodies, unlike my mother did with me—but then again it was a very different time back then. I'm so happy that topics such as 'the change' can be talked about freely now rather than be a taboo subject.

. . . ask what makes you come alive, and go do that because what the world needs are people who have come alive. What pleasure invites us to it, what makes us come alive in our bodies? What makes us light up? What makes us activate? Because in that activation is the ability, is the stamina to change the world.[3]

Sonya Renee Taylor

CHAPTER 12

Queen Menopause

What a crazy ride this hormonal journey has been. I think about where I was as a young girl starting her cycle. The young woman afraid to speak, to protect herself. Finding herself standing in the spotlight of fame. The wife that felt unworthy of love. The young mum who was so naive.

Time spent in therapy, digging in and digging up old beliefs, old patterns. Neglecting to take care of myself as I nurtured my children, my job and those around me. The crashing of my health and moving countries. Then to perimenopause.

If there is one common theme throughout my life, it's been about learning to love myself for exactly who I am. The idea that if only I looked great in a two-piece bikini, that if I didn't have the wrinkles or stretch marks, *then* I could love myself more is such a load of bullshit, because I *did* have all that and a bag of chips. I had magazine covers, I had articles heralding me as 'the perfect woman'. All that adoration, and I still didn't feel I loved who I was.

I'm now getting the message. I was a little slow, I know . . . You know the one about it's not how you look but how you feel?

Though it's so much more.

It's realising women are outrageously amazing. Complex, strong, brave. We carry so much within our bodies—all the stories, all the pain, all the joy

So honestly, we (and that includes me) really need to give ourselves a goddamn break.

The heroine's journey

You might have heard of something called, 'the hero's journey'. It's the basis of a story about an ordinary person who goes on a quest, finds adventure and challenges and returns changed. Every Pixar movie is based on this theme; in fact, so many books and movies follow this roadmap of sorts.

Many people resonate with the hero's journey as it gives us a feeling that meaningful transformation is possible. It shows us that we can overcome our inner and outer obstacles, become stronger and win the day.

In thinking about the hero's journey, I can't help but make the link between a woman's experience and how connected it is to the same path, or, as I like to call it, 'the heroine's journey'.

1 *Ordinary world*

Here we are as women, just keeping up to speed with life in general. All might be well, no aches or pains, and sleep is taken for granted. We might be ticking all the boxes that our younger selves dreamed we would: marriage, career, kids, no kids, travel.

2 *Call to adventure*

But wait, there are rumblings about. We begin to hear other women speak of hot flushes, and other disturbances. The word perimenopause is lightly thrown around. Haha! But no, what of this perimenopause? You don't need to be thinking of such things yet, or do you? Is there a new challenge laid before you? One that no one has yet explained?

3 *Refusal of the call*

At first we deny: I'm too young. No, this must be something else. Can't be perimenopause yet. But maybe it is. Or maybe it's just a phase, stress at work interrupting your sleep, summer making you feel extra hot, cycle changing—must just be this month. So, you're a little more emotional this week, that's normal too, right? Can't be perimenopause.

4 *Meeting the mentor*

But more changes seem to be happening. We start to broach the subject of menopause with other women, we hear their stories of what lies ahead. Some symptoms have you worried. Women older than you are postmenopausal; they mention this 'zest'. Our concerns have been put to rest . . . for now.

5 *Crossing the threshold*

It's been months now of rising symptoms, sleep is elusive, moods are up and down. Random aches are presenting themselves and relationships are feeling strained. We begin to look at the ways that we need to take better care of ourselves, and seek joy not in what we look like but who we are—how we spend our time is precious to us. We make a commitment to be healthier, eat better, take extra walks and maybe even slow down.

6 *Tests, allies, enemies*

The enemy. The mirror and the judging voice inside our heads. What do I see in the mirror but lines and a roll of fat that was not there six months ago? Judgement kicks in, self-doubt creeps into our world. The reflection is something we don't like and we feel the sadness and loss of our youth. We learn not to trust in the view of ourselves when we are in a negative mind space. We look to friends to assist us through this time.

7 *Approach to the inmost cave*

Our skin may itch, our hair may change, our mind may fog. We wrestle with what we 'should feel' and what we don't, we may feel that no one understands what we have lost, and we look backward at the wonder of our past. Though we turn inwards, we know our power and beauty. We feel the approach of something different.

8 *Ordeal*

And summer arrives. Cue more hot flushes and bikini season. Change room, trying on swimsuits. Overhead lighting. Next size up, please. Still, we set foot on the beach and we march to the water's edge to bravely dive in, understanding that it's how the water makes you feel: the fresh tang of the salt, the sand between your toes. And that no one is judging you but yourself.

9 *Reward (seizing the sword)*

So now the reward for speaking more kindly to yourself. After defeating the enemy, which is your own judgement, your inner critic. After overcoming your greatest personal challenge—you realise you are reborn, you have emerged as a stronger, smarter, wiser woman, capable of so many things.

10 *The road back*

So now you return home to yourself, making peace with all the changes big and small. You speak and share your challenges and triumphs. Hot flushes have waned, your body feels like yours again. Sleep beckons once more.

11 *Resurrection*

This is the moment you do not allow anyone outside of yourself to define you. You are visible, you embrace your age, your body. You must, for there are others in your wake who are looking to see how you've anchored in the changes you've experienced. You tell others to not be afraid and to share in the joy that you've gained from all that you have learned along the way.

12 Return with the elixir

Final stage. You now bring fresh hope to those around you. You are in celebration of who you are. Periods, gone. Judgement, gone. Caring what others think, gone. Intimacy with your partner, back. Health, fitness, back. The elixir is YOU.

—

Journal entry, May 2020

Feeling lighter, stronger today than I have in a while. I literally feel the spring in my step. Can catch the scent of possibilities in the wind. What do I want to do with the rest of my life, my days here on earth? I feel capable of so much right now. I feel my relationship with my friends deepening. I am tracking the ways I still feel stuck around speaking up and I take a deep breath, centring myself, I feel less afraid of telling my truth. I feel much more comfortable with what I have and how I spend my time and with whom. I feel so grateful for the people around me, the people cheering me on, the people who tell me I can do it, that I am strong and brave. I see my children owning their independence as I own mine.

—

I've been on the road to wholeness since I first started working with a therapist. Sometimes I've taken three steps forward and two steps back. Sometimes I've spent far too much time analysing every darn small thing I say or do.

Finally feeling the freedom of my words and letting go of this idea that I can't please everyone have been liberating.

I'm still rescuing myself from the expectations about women and how we are supposed to look and act. I'm finding the balance by shaking my fist at mainstream ideas of how I'm supposed to dress.

I wrote this book to tear the chains off myself. I've been locked up with suppressed anger and a lack of self-worth for so long. Not trusting myself and the wisdom I've accrued over the years. I still find my people pleaser wants to take over, though less and less. I still have a battle with how I look in the mirror, though again, I'm much more likely to say, 'Fuck it, you're gorgeous,' these days more than ever.

Looking ahead I want more: more of me, my voice. I want to stand in the body I have now and see and feel the beauty that is me. I want to be brave with my life and choices, to not care what strangers think of me. I want to not only be present in the moment, but look forward to my life ahead. I want to be an uplifting person, not only to myself and the people around me, but for women who need a voice to cheer them on. I want to catch the shit I hurl at myself and turn it into kindness. I want to grow alongside my husband and continue to create a life that exemplifies joy and gratitude to our kids. I want to redefine making love with him.

And when the time comes, I want to be the coolest, funkiest, funniest, most compassionate, loving grandma around.

I want to always speak my mind, say my truth and protect myself and others.

I understand that sometimes I need to look into the empty spaces of my life to understand what it is that I *do* want.

Menopause has taught me a lot about emptiness, and some of the lessons have been painful. The ones where I can't have my children as babes in arms again, or feel the excitement of a pregnancy and all that a new life entails. So many 'first times' for this or that. It's more challenging to find 'first times' now. Though I'm more aware than ever that I need to seek them out. First time writing a book!

I've never been so confronted by my beliefs about who I am and how I treat myself than when going through menopause. I've found myself at the beginning of writing this book at a crossroads. A mid-life crisis, to use that turn of phrase. What am I going to do with all these feelings, physical pains and changes, these writhing emotions and this exploding anger?

How do I live within my old life while so many things are falling apart? When am I going to start loving who I am?

I never expected any of these questions to arise, though here they are. I hear them when I see my reflection in my mirror. That nasty girl was allowed to run rampant in my brain for too long, judging every nook and cranny, every misstep I made. Now I have someone on my side: me.

I really need that voice; she's been silenced for far too long.

Life does give you lemons, because she knows you can make something delicious with them if you just trust that you can. All my experiences, from girl to womanhood to mother and now midlife, have built me a foundation that I can call on when I need to. I absolutely have more to change, more to speak up about, but I feel freer to do so.

I hope that you do, too.

This is a book of discoveries, about trying to explain the insides and the outsides of myself. It's doing justice to my life without trying to denigrate myself in order to be liked by you, the reader. I've spent a lifetime making sure everyone else is okay with who I am and not making sure *I* am okay with who I am. Menopause and aging have finally shifted this dynamic for me.

Can I make menopause cool and a trending hashtag? #muffintopsarein? #hotwomenflush Highly unlikely. But how about we begin to see ourselves as Queen Menopause? Yes, my sceptre might be my handheld fan, but why not own this title, this crown?

When I look back, I think about everything that has led me here. We all begin again every day; every time we wake up it's another renewal. So goes menopause—it's a renewal of the most significant kind. A metamorphosis involving some mighty big changes. If we didn't experience all the changes and pains and challenges, would the other side of it feel as sweet? I think not. The most beautiful sunset is from the top of the mountain you climbed yourself. So keep climbing, make sure you take your crown. You earned it.

You are Queen Menopause.

Thank you for reading my story. Please go tell yours; tell it with all the feelings and emotion it deserves, the tears and rage, the sadness and loneliness—tell it all, because not only will it help you, but it just might help someone else tell theirs. Let's take menopause out of the shadows, learn about what it means for us and then keep taking steps to our next destination. Whatever those steps may be for you, I hope they're filled with laughter, beauty, creativity, joy, acceptance and most importantly love. Go gently with yourself.

When she started letting go, her vision became clearer. The present felt more manageable and the future began to look open and full of bright possibilities. As she shed the tense energy of the past, her creativity and power returned to her. With a revitalized excitement, she focused on building a new life where joy and freedom were abundant.

Yung Pueblo
....

Journal entry, July 2020

Here I am today, the craziest year, and I feel . . . good. I woke up and realised I no longer feel the grief of not being fertile, not being able to make babies; I no longer feel that the best part of my life is behind me. I'm not walking on a tightrope of moods. The headaches I was experiencing have gone, the hot flushes have waned to only one or two a day and are far less deadly than when they first started. Even in a world gone nuts with a pandemic and political upheaval my 3 a.m. conspiracy theories have thankfully shut the hell up. Whenever I post something on my Instagram relating to menopause, the outpouring of comments around this subject lets me know I am not alone, that we need each other and that women supporting women is just about the most beautiful experience there is. I love my husband, I am so grateful that I love my husband. That all that chatter, that pushing to find fault, the snapping, has removed itself and I can see him clearly again. My skin has settled, too, it's no longer itchy or dry. The self-love journey will continue for me for sure. I'm not at a full year yet since my last period, so I can't say I'm postmenopausal.

Though I'm so close, and I'm so excited. I'm through the toughest part and I'm planning on sliding into home base and joining the team of fabulous women who are cheering me on from the bleachers.

Acknowledgements

This book was written over three years and one pandemic. It never would have existed without the lovely Claire Kingston. I had been pondering a book on menopause for just a few weeks when out of the blue a simple line on my Instagram bio, 'Menopausal mother of three', caught her attention and she floated the idea of the book. I thank the whole Allen & Unwin team, especially the ever-so-awesome Jane Palfreyman, for supporting the book and propping up my ego when I thought the book was basically a pile of crap. The wonderful Samantha Kent, who has the patience of a saint answering all my first-time author questions. The editor, Angela Meyer, who saw the book in its most rough form and created sense of it. The fabulous typesetters at Bookhouse, who did one last flourish and added a sprinkle of magic.

Thank you.

My family, my two sisters Karen and Mell, who have watched the weird and curvy, wild and woolly, crazy highs and super lows of my life and careers and still love me. I love you both. My beautiful mum, whose love and kindness wrap me up like a warm hug every time I hear your voice and see your face. And especially my dad, who I remember, as a kid, watching for hours on the lounge room floor proofreading your own books. I still think you have another book in you!

You're an inspiration. Thank you for all the love.

To my gang of ladies in America, who I painfully left behind, all of you—each and every single one—have shaped me, supported me and loved me through thick and thin. The Marco Polos with you, Susan Grace, continue to be a highlight. ☺

A special shout out to Carrie Anne Moss who said years ago, well before my first symptom of perimenopause, 'I see you writing a book and creating retreats for women going through menopause'.

I thought you were nuts.

All of the women and men in this book, Traci, Maria, Anita, Neeyah, Louise and Ken, Sally, Rhonda, Georgie, Lynne, Anita Heiss and Cam, thank you from the bottom of my heart for your generous time and honesty—your stories are so much of the heart and soul of the book.

Everyone needs a champion while tackling a first-time challenging job. I'm so fortunate to have one. She came in with guns blazing and her whip-smart mind ready to listen, read and cheer me through the times when I was absolutely lost. Claire Weir, thank you is not a big enough word for our walks together, your time, your humour, your editing and support—I would have been seriously lost without you. Did I mention to you that I'm a high school dropout?

Carlotta Moye, you've been with me for some mighty big times in my life: my modelling career, meeting Cam, as my bridesmaid. You were the only person I truly trusted with the photograph for the cover of this book. Thank you for your creative spirit and your gorgeous soul.

Cathy Baker, my agent who is just an all-round amazing human, your support in reading the book once in its early, rough form gave me such a kick in the pants to keep going—thank you for everything.

Dr Rebecca Ray—Bec—thank you for our Instagram friendship that turned into a stream of support and delight. Your knowledge of first-time book writing and talking me down off the edge were much appreciated. You're an angel.

Thank you to all the women so much wiser than me who are already living a beautiful, bountiful wonderful juicy life. Your light shines bright for other women like me to follow.

People always leave the most special people till last in these thank yous. I can hear the drum roll as I begin to write my biggest and most shiny thank you to my family: Lotus, River, Bodhi and, of course, Cam. I adore you all. Not only have you supported and encouraged me to keep writing, but you also had to experience menopause with me. To my girls, I hope you have a copy of this book when you are older, I hope you open and read it then and think, *hey this actually helps me*. I hope you understand your mum a little better as well, but mostly I hope you move through your menopause with love and grace. Cam—my partner, friend, cheerleader, bedfellow, best barbequeing husband ever. Thank you for everything, mostly for your excitement about this book especially the times when I couldn't find it in myself. Thank you for listening and listening and listening to me talk about menopause. Maybe now we are even, you with golf talk, me with menopause talk. I love you.

Notes

Chapter 2

1 '10 "fun" facts about menopause', Gransnet, www.gransnet.com/health/
menopause-facts-treatments

Chapter 4

1 Lisa Rapaport, 'Culture may influence how women experience menopause',
Reuters, 6 June 2015, www.reuters.com/article/us-health-menopause-perceptions/
culture-may-influence-how-women-experience-menopause-
idUSKBN0OL1XH20150605

2 Brené Brown, 'Shame vs. Guilt', 15 January 2013, brenebrown.com/
blog/2013/01/14/shame-v-guilt/

3 Tracee Ellis Ross, 'A woman's fury holds lifetimes of wisdom', April 2018, www.
ted.com/talks/tracee_ellis_ross_a_woman_s_fury_holds_lifetimes_of_wisdom

4 Christiane Northrup, 'Women's Wisdom versus Patriarchal Programming', 18
March 2014, www.drnorthrup.com/womens-wisdom-versus-patriarchal-
programming/

Chapter 6

1   Pauline Porizkova, 'Aging', *HuffPost*, The Blog, 21 October 2010, www.huffpost.
    com/entry/aging_b_771127
2   Laurie Meyers, 'Falling short of perfect', Counseling Today, 28 March 2018,
    ct.counseling.org/2016/03/falling-short-of-perfect

Chapter 7

1   Nancy Schimelpfening, 'Why Depression Is More Common in Women Than in
    Men', verywellmind, 24 December 2020, www.verywellmind.com/why-is-
    depression-more-common-in-women-1067040
2   Dr Josh Axe, 'Menopause Symptoms to Watch For and Ways to Relieve Them',
    Dr. Axe, 26 October 2018, draxe.com/health/relieve-your-menopause-symptoms/

Chapter 8

1   Janine Shepherd, facebook, 10 December 2019, facebook.com/
    janineshepherdauthor/photos/when-we-share-our-stories-we-open-our-hearts-to-
    allow-others-to-share-their-stor/2578486205533154/
2   Eric Berlin MD, 'Your Menopause Experience May Depend on Your Cultural
    Background', Everyday Health, 10 February 2009, www.everydayhealth.com/
    menopause/menopause-and-culture.aspx
3   Ibid.
4   Jamie Lee Curtis, 'Anti-Anti', *HuffPost*, 22 May 2012, www.huffpost.com/entry/
    against-anti-aging_b_1372366
5   Hilary Osborne and Caroline Bannock, '"I miss what I used to be like": women's
    stories of the menopause', *Guardian*, 26 August 2019, theguardian.com/society/2019/
    aug/25/i-miss-what-i-used-to-be-like-womens-stories-of-the-menopause
6   Cathy Garrard, 'Coping With Hot Flashes and Other Menopausal Symptoms:
    What Celebrities Said', Everyday Health, 22 February 2021, www.everydayhealth.
    com/menopause/coping-hot-flashes-menopausal-symptoms-celebrities-said/

Chapter 9

1   Jane Gardner, 'Acupuncture treats hot flushes—but there's a catch', Pursuit,
    University of Melbourne, first published 19 January 2016 in Health and Wellbeing,
    pursuit.unimelb.edu.au/articles/acupuncture-treats-hot-flushes-but-there-s-a-
    catch

2   Laila Ahmed Abou Ismail et al., 'Effect of Acupuncture on Body Weight Reduction and Inflammatory Mediators in Egyptian Obese Patients', Open Access Maced J Med Sci, www.ncbi.nlm.nih.gov/pmc/articles/PMC4877795/

3   Dr John Axe, 'What is adrenal fatigue? Steps to overcome it naturally', Dr Axe, 2 April 2021, draxe.com/3-steps-to-heal-adrenal-fatigue/

4   Gunver S. Kienle, et al., 'Anthroposophic Medicine: An Integrative Medical System Originating in Europe', Glob Adv Health Med., vol. 2, no, 6, November 2013, pp. 20–31, www.ncbi.nlm.nih.gov/pmc/articles/PMC3865373/

5   Nadia Marshall, Mudita Institute & Health Clinic, www.muditainstitute.com

6   T. Shams et al., 'Efficacy of black cohosh-containing preparations on menopausal symptoms', Database of Abstracts of Reviews of Effects (DARE), Centre for Reviews and Dissemination (UK), 1995, www.ncbi.nlm.nih.gov/books/NBK79338

7   K. Jiang et al, 'Black cohosh improves objective sleep in postmenopausal women with sleep disturbance', Climacteric, vol, 1, no, 4, pp., 559–67, 22 May 2015, www.pubmed.ncbi.nlm.nih.gov/26000551/

8   Gita, 'Sore Breasts? Best ways to reduce menopause Breast Tenderness', My Menopause Journey', mymenopausejourney.com/breast-tenderness-menopause/

9   http://thinkoily.com/essential-oils-for-hot-flashes-night-sweats. Accessed 2021.

10 '6 Essential Oils for Menopause Relief', Cure Joy, 28 march 2017, www.curejoy.com/content/essential-oils-for-menopause/

11 Kate Bracy, 'Benefits of Vitamin D for Women in Menopause', verywellhealth,18 May 2021, www.verywellhealth.com/vitamin-d-your-prevention-ally-2322660

12 Cathy Wong, 'Evening Primrose Oil and Menopause', verywellhealth, 30 April 2020, www.verywellhealth.com/evening-primrose-and-menopause-90067

13 Blog, '10 Nutrients for Healthy Hair During Menopause', www.mariongluckclinic.com/blog/nutrients-healthy-hair-menopause.html

14 Christiane Northrup, 'Heart Palpitations: A Message from your Midlife Heart', 2012, www.drnorthrup.com/palpitations-a-message-from-your-midlife-heart/

15 Agi Mary Joseph, 'Hormone imbalance in women and Homeopathy', Holistic Homeopathy Brisbane, 5 July 2019, holistichomeopathy.com.au/blog/hormonal-imbalance-in-woman-and-homeopathy

16 'What is HRT?', You and Your Hormones, May 2021, www.yourhormones.info/topical-issues/what-is-hrt/

17 www.fergon.com/what-to-know-about-perimenopause-iron-deficiency/. Accessed 2021.

18 Cindy Joseph, 'Hadley's Story', Boom!, 3 May 2019, www.boombycindyjoseph.com/blogs/boom/hadleys-story

19   'Can menopause cause itching? Tips for relief', Medical News Today, www.medicalnewstoday.com/articles/322587#home-remedies

20   'Joint Pain', Australian Menopause Centre, www.menopausecentre.com.au/joint-pain

21   Blog, Dr Happy, www.drhappy.com.au/blog/

22   '9 Best Essential Oils for Menopause', Essential Oil Sanctuary, essentialoilsanctuary.com/menopause/

23   Lara Briden, '8 Ways that Magnesium Rescues Hormones', 30 March 2014, www.larabriden.com/8-ways-that-magnesium-rescues-hormones/

24   Ellen Dolgen, 'Menopause Meditation Tips', ellendolgen.com/2021/11/menopause-meditation-tips/

25   'How Omega-e Can Provide Relief for Menopausal Symptoms', Australian Menopause Centre, menopausecentre.com.au/information-centre/articles/how-omega-3-can-provide-relief-for-menopausal-symptoms/

26   See '9 Best Essential Oils for Menopause' above

27   Suzie Skwiot, 'What Teas Help with Menopause Symptoms Relief', Healthline, 9 February 2022, www.healthline.com/health/menopause/tea-for-menopause#teas-for-relief

28   Christiane Northrup, 'Menopause', www.drnorthrup.com/category/health/womens-wisdom/menopause/

29   'Oprah & Deepak 21 day meditation experience', chopracentermeditation.com/article/6-oprah_deepaks_21_day_ meditation_experience

30   'Herbal Remedies Traditionally Used for Treating Menopause', Australian Menopause Centre, www.menopausecentre.com.au/information-centre/articles/herbal-remedies-for-treating-menopause/

31   Chris Feytag, 'The Hidden Ingredient Making Your Menopause Symptoms Worse', Get Healthy, 29 December 2016, gethealthyu.com/ingredient-making-your-menopause-symptoms-worse/. Accessed 2021

32   Shruti, '11 Ways Turmeric Benefits in Menopause and Post-Menopause', www.turmericforhealth.com/turmeric-benefits/11-ways-turmeric-can-help-in-menopause-and-post-menopause

33   Naturally Daily Team, '10 Effective Home Remedies for Vaginal Dryness', 25 June 2019, naturallydaily.com/home-remedies-for-vaginal-dryness/

34   Cheryl MacDonald, 'Yoga for menopause—7 reasons why it's great', The Mutton Club, themuttonclub.com/yoga-for-symptoms-of-menopause/

35   Magdalena Wszelaki, 'Using the Mighty Zinc to Balance Your Hormones', Hormones & Balance, 10 march 2021, hormonesbalance.com/articles/using-the-mighty-zinc-to-balance-your-hormones/

36   Amy Froneman, 'Zisyphus may be the answer to a natural night's sleep', Health 24, 3 July 2014, www.news24.com/health24/Medical/Sleep/treating-sleep-problems/Zizyphus-as-a-sleep-aid-20140703

Chapter 10

1   '8 Ways Perimenopause Actually Makes Life Better, From Women Who've Been There', First for Women, 20 November 2018, www.firstforwomen.com/posts/health/perimenopause-benefits-163417
2   Dr Josh Axe, 'Menopause Symptoms to Watch for and Ways to Relieve Them', Dr. Axe, 26 October 2018, https://draxe.com/health/relieve-your-menopause-symptoms/
3   Ed Yong, 'Why Killer Whales Go Through Menopause But Elephants Don't', *National Geographic*, 4 March 2015, www.nationalgeographic.com/science/article/why-killer-whales-go-through-menopause-but-elephants-dont

Chapter 11

1   Brené Brown, 'Own Our History, Change the Story', 18 June 2015, brenebrown.com/blog/2015/06/18/own-our-history-change-the-story/
2   Anita Heiss, *Tiddas*, Simon & Schuster, Sydney, 2014
3   Brené Brown, 'Brené with Sonya Renee Taylor on "The Body is Not An Apology"', Thisten, https://thisten.co/tr53q/G9Um1orcbEMlT2ievwb4W5HgtEaV30KJgShn0dTg